For Reasons of Legality

ISBN: 0-9767944-8-9

Published by Ener-Chi Wellness Press (Ener-chi.com), U.S.A.
June 2006
Cover Design/Artwork (Ener-chi Art, Oil on Canvas): By Andreas Moritz

Simple Steps
to
Total Health

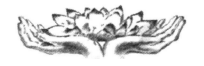

Your Health is in Your Hands

Also by Andreas Moritz
. . .

**The Amazing Liver
& Gallbladder Flush**

**Timeless Secrets of
Health & Rejuvenation**

Lifting the Veil of Duality

Cancer Is Not A Disease (New)

Heart Disease No More

It's Time to Come Alive

The Art of Self Healing
(End of 2006)

Sacred Santémony

Ener-Chi Art

Ener-Chi 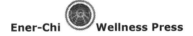 **Wellness Press**

Acknowledgment

The authors would like to express their deep gratitude to Lillian S. Maresch for her skillful editing, creative ideas and inspiration.

Table of Contents

Preface

Over the past three decades, as I provided health consultations to thousands of clients in various countries throughout the world, I have been creating a continually expanding series of books that present important information on a wide range of health issues. For a person who is in the early stages of taking responsibility for their own health, this library of information can seem a bit overwhelming. Consequently, I have often been asked to develop some simple guidelines to serve as a starting point for those in quest of better health. This book is intended to respond to those requests.

The guidelines and suggestions provided here can have a profound impact on the health of anyone who is willing to take them seriously, and make the corresponding changes in their personal hygiene, diet and lifestyle. For those who want to delve into certain subjects in greater depth, I have included references to other books and resources that contain more detailed information.

Andreas Moritz
(May 21, 2006)

Introduction

Health and vitality are the natural states of being for the human body. Because of eating habits and lifestyle choices, however, most people are suffering from various health conditions that inhibit their ability to enjoy life to the fullest. Unfortunately, the predominant medical approach is to treat such situations with medication or surgery that may provide temporary relief for the symptoms, but virtually never correct the root cause of the problem. It is becoming increasingly apparent that the side effects of such medical practices are often more damaging to our health than the original ailment.

"Iatrogenic" is the medical term for illnesses that are caused by the medical profession. It is difficult to obtain accurate information on the extent of this problem because of potential litigation issues. However, a 10 year study[17] of government statistics completed in 2003 concluded that iatrogenic illness is now the *leading* cause of death in the United States. And further, it concluded that adverse reactions to prescription drugs are responsible for more that 300,000 deaths each year. That is the equivalent of more than two full jumbo jets falling out of the sky every day!

The intent here is not to criticize the millions of dedicated medical practitioners, most of whom are working long hours every day in an effort to relieve the pain and suffering of patients who are in need. Rather, it is to suggest that the western medical model that relies primarily on medication and surgery has taken a wrong turn.

It is up to each of us to learn how to care for our own body. Unfortunately, most of the information with which we are bombarded on a daily basis is provided by companies who are interested in selling us products or providing us services, rather than helping us understand how to keep our bodies healthy. The human body has amazing resiliency and recuperative powers. If we work in cooperation with the natural functioning of the body, it is seldom too late to make changes that will enable us to begin our journey on the road to full healing and rejuvenation.

The human body is not just a physical mechanism; it is a complex unit that also involves our thoughts, emotions and spiritual nature. The purpose of this book is to provide a few basics on how the human body functions, and to offer suggestions, including lifestyle considerations, on how each of us can care for our body in a way that will promote optimum health and longevity.

Part 1

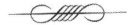

The Most Common Causes of Disease

"Internal Hygiene"

The most common causes of disease all relate to a build-up of toxins and residues in the body that inhibit the various organs and systems from performing their normal functions. We may think of this in terms of *internal hygiene*.

As children, most of us were taught to regularly wash our hands and face, brush our teeth, wash our hair, and bathe or take a shower – all aspects of *external* hygiene. Unfortunately, most of us were never taught the importance or the methods of *internal* hygiene – keeping our internal organs and systems clean and well hydrated.

Our cultural attitude is that the best we can hope for is a reasonably healthy childhood and early adulthood. Nevertheless, as we progress into middle age and eventually our later years, the expectation is that our health, vitality and mobility will gradually deteriorate. We tend to think that our only option is to slow down the deterioration as much as possible. Unfortunately, if we resort to medications or surgery in response to various symptoms of illness within the body, we only tend to exacerbate the problem.

Most of us have never been taught about the regenerative powers of the body – that if we work in harmony with the natural processes of the body, cleaning out the toxins and residues as they accumulate, and making appropriate changes to our eating and lifestyle habits, the vitality and mobility that we experienced in our younger years can be restored. Even if we are approaching the twilight years of life, it is virtually never too late to reverse the trend of deteriorating health.

Each of the four chapters in Part 1 focuses on a particular aspect of internal hygiene and hydration of the body, but they are all closely interrelated. If one chooses to go through the various cleansing and hydration processes that are recommended, it is important to follow the guidelines that are provided so that the toxins are removed in a gradual, properly sequenced, and safe manner. Otherwise, a toxicity crisis could be created, endangering the health of the body.

Chapter 1

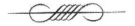

Congestion within the Liver and Gallbladder

The liver, which is the largest organ in the body, is responsible for processing, distributing and maintaining the body's "fuel supply." Also, it makes new amino acids and converts existing ones into proteins, which serve as building blocks for every cell in the body. Another function of the liver is to break down alcohol and other toxic substances, including bacteria, parasites and certain drug compounds. As more than a quart of blood is filtered through the liver every minute, toxins are removed and nutrients are distributed throughout the body.

Yet another important role of the liver is to produce bile, which is crucial to the proper digestion of food. The gallbladder functions in conjunction with the liver, serving primarily as a reservoir for the bile that is produced in the liver. Bile is produced at a fairly constant rate throughout the day. However, the need for bile varies in accordance with the digestive cycles. During periods of peak demand, bile flow from the liver is supplemented by bile that has been stored the gallbladder.

One of the most common health problems involves the formation of hardened "stones" within the liver and gallbladder. These stones are usually referred to as "gallstones" when they occur in the gallbladder, and "intrahepatic" or "biliary" stones when they occur in the liver (see **Figures 1 & 2**). However, since most stones of both types are of a similar nature, they will be referred to in this book as "gallstones," regardless of whether they reside in the gallbladder or liver.

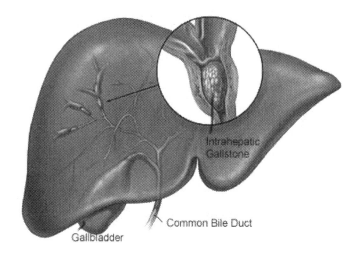

Intrahepatic Gallstone

Common Bile Duct

Gallbladder

Figure 1: (Intrahepatic) Gallstones in the Liver Bile Ducts

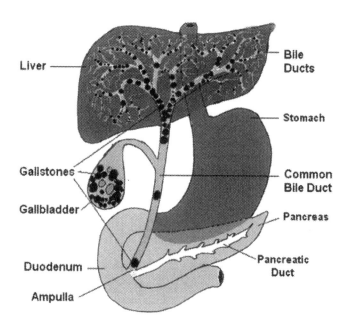

Liver

Bile Ducts

Stomach

Gallstones

Gallbladder

Common Bile Duct

Pancreas

Duodenum

Pancreatic Duct

Ampulla

Figure 2: Gallstones in the Liver and Gallbladder

Gallstones form because of an unhealthy diet and/or lifestyle. They consist primarily of cholesterol and other residues. In a chronic situation, it is not uncommon for a person's liver and gallbladder to contain as many as several thousand gallstones, ranging from approximately the size of a grain of wheat, to that of a pea. However, they occasionally grow considerably larger. When the liver and gallbladder become congested with gallstones, all of the functions of the liver become impaired. Most commonly, the gallstones become lodged in the bile ducts and inhibit the flow of bile to the digestive tract. In severe cases, the amount of bile reaching the digestive tract may be only 25% of that which is needed for proper digestion.

Gallstones also interfere with the detoxification processes that normally take place within the liver. Over time, as the blood vessels within the liver become increasingly clogged, the normal flow of blood through the liver, and the consequent distribution of nutrients through the body, becomes restricted.

Symptoms of congestion within the liver and gallbladder due to gallstones can be many and varied. Some examples are:

- Chronic fatigue
- Headaches and migraines
- Digestive disorders
- Constipation
- Diarrhea
- Aches and pains in the joints
- Shoulder, neck & back pain
- Food cravings
- High cholesterol
- Obesity
- Skin disorders and discoloration
- Depression
- Sexual impotence
- Urinary problems
- Menstrual and menopausal disorders

- Tooth and gum problems
- Osteoporosis
- Cancer
- Difficulty sleeping
- Cold extremities
- Allergies

Liver and Gallbladder Flush

The good news is that gallstones can be removed from the liver and gallbladder through a rather simple series of cleanses. And by maintaining a healthy diet and lifestyle, most, if not all, of the symptoms will begin to disappear. Almost invariably, there will be a noticeable increase in one's energy level even after just the first cleanse.

Information on how to do a liver cleanse is available in the book, *The Amazing Liver and Gallbladder Flush.*[16]

It is interesting to note that with health care costs in the United States now exceeding $1.6 *trillion* annually, the single most important thing we can do to restore and maintain health and vitality – a liver and gallbladder flush – can be done at home with items readily available in groceries for a cost of about $10.

Chapter 2

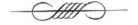

Dehydration

Dehydration of the body is one of the most common health problems. Drinking sufficient quantities of water at appropriate times throughout the day is probably the single most important thing we can do to improve our health.[1] Perhaps this is not surprising when we realize that about 75% of our body consists of water.

Virtually all of the organs and systems within the human body require adequate amounts of water in order to function properly. People who do not drink enough water gradually lower the ratio of the volume of water that exists inside the cells, to the volume of water that is found outside the cells. This undermines all cellular activity, whether it involves cells of the skin, stomach, liver, kidneys, heart or brain.

Whenever there is cellular dehydration, metabolic waste products are not removed properly. This causes symptoms that resemble disease. Since more and more of the water within the body begins to accumulate outside the cells, this may typically manifest as water retention within the feet, legs, arms and face. Consequently, dehydration may not be apparent to the afflicted person. In addition, the kidneys may begin to hold on to water, markedly reducing urinary secretion, and causing retention of potentially harmful waste products within the body.

Normally, cellular enzymes signal the brain when cells run out of water. However, enzymes in dehydrated cells become so inefficient that they are no longer able to register the drought-like conditions, and consequently fail to push the "thirst alarm button" within the brain.

A dehydrated person may also be suffering from lack of energy. Under normal conditions, the water we drink keeps the cell volume balanced and the salt we eat maintains the balanced volume of water that is kept outside the cells and in circulation. This generates the proper osmotic pressure necessary for cellular nourishment and energy production. During dehydration, this basic mechanism begins to fail, leading to loss of energy and potentially serious cell damage.

Another major indicator of dehydration in the body is pain. In response to a shortage of water, the brain activates and stores the important neurotransmitter, *histamine*. In turn, the histamine directs subordinate water regulators to redistribute the water to areas where it is needed for essential metabolic and survival activity. When histamine and its subordinate regulators come across pain-sensing nerves in the body, they trigger strong and continual pain. These pain signals may manifest, for example, as rheumatoid arthritis, angina, low back problems or headaches.

Drinking Water - The Greatest Therapy of All

Drinking a sufficient amount of fresh water is an essential prerequisite for avoiding disease and slowing the aging process. Anyone who is relatively healthy and wants to stay that way needs to drink approximately 6 to 8 glasses (8 oz. per glass) of water each day. This will ensure that the body maintains a sufficient level of hydration, which is necessary for efficient digestion, metabolism and waste removal. Our water intake should be adjusted to take into account body weight, with larger bodies needing proportionately more water. In addition, exercise and other activities that stimulate perspiration create a need for additional water.

Suggested Tips & Schedule

- *Start the day by drinking one glass of warm water. This will end the "drought" resulting from not drinking fluids*

8

during the relatively long period of sleep during the night and remove accumulated wastes from the excretory organs. Follow this with a second glass of warm water enhanced with the juice from a wedge of lemon and a teaspoon of honey. The addition of lemon and honey has a very cleansing effect on the body (the amount of lemon juice may be increased if desired).

- *About half an hour before each meal, drink one glass of water. Doing this will keep your blood thin and help it to take in all the nutrients your cells need to function efficiently. The water also helps increase the secretion of digestive juices, which improves the digestion of food. In contrast, drinking a lot of water or other beverages with your meal dilutes the digestive juices, which greatly undermines the digestive process and can lead to weight gain.*

- *Following a meal, the blood uses up a considerable amount of water to distribute nutrients to the cells. In effect, the blood can become water deficient quite quickly. To counteract this, drink a glass of water approximately 2-3 hours after breakfast and lunch to restore the blood's water requirements (this is not as necessary in the evening, given the naturally slow digestion and physical activity at this time of day).*

Water Quality

Ideally, the water we drink should be some form of natural spring water or artesian water. Most city or community water systems treat the water with chemicals, such as chlorine, to kill the bacteria. Of course, the ingested chlorine also kills the beneficial bacteria that are responsible for helping us digest our food. Chlorinated water causes havoc in our body and is responsible for countless illnesses. Fluoride in drinking water is just has harmful. Therefore, tap water should be filtered to remove these chemicals before it is consumed. Fortunately, there are many different types of water filters that are now commercially available and relatively inexpensive.

Also, it is best to drink water that is at room temperature or slightly warmer. Ice water tends to constrict the muscles in the digestive tract, preventing them from functioning properly. Iced beverages also numb the nerve endings in the stomach, thereby inhibiting balanced acid secretions. If ice water is the only water available, it is best to drink it one swallow at a time, holding it in the mouth to warm it up somewhat before swallowing it. Ice served in restaurants has recently been found to contain more bacteria than toilet water.

An Important Note of Caution

Restoring proper hydration in the body should be done gradually, otherwise it could have harmful consequences! During severe dehydration, the body's cells are not able to function efficiently. To protect themselves against further loss of water, the cells make their membranes less penetrable to water diffusion by pulling in extra amounts of fats, including cholesterol. In this condition, it would be unwise to suddenly start drinking large quantities of water. Since the cells have created a barrier in order to save water, they are in no position to absorb increased water all at once. The water would simply stagnate outside the cells and lead to water retention and weight gain.

Also, during dehydration the kidneys hold on to water, as does the rest of the body. When this happens, many people start craving and overeating salt or salty foods because the body needs more salt to retain the small amount of water it has. This, however, causes the kidneys to tighten and filter even less water, and the urine becomes more and more concentrated. Under these conditions, the kidneys are not able to filter much urine, and any sudden intake of large amounts of water can cause severe lymph congestion, swelling, and in extreme cases, even death.

The transition from a state of severe dehydration to improved hydration should be very gradual and is best monitored by a health practitioner who understands the basics of water metabolism.

Dangers Inherent in Common Beverages

In most modern cultures, the majority of people tend to respond to the body's natural thirst signal by drinking beverages such as coffee, tea, soft drinks, beer, wine, or a wide range of other concoctions. While it is true that such drinks contain water, they also contain other things such as caffeine, alcohol, sugar, artificial sweeteners or other chemicals that act as strong dehydrators. The more of these beverages one consumes, the more dehydrated the body becomes. The effects they create in the body are exactly the opposite to the ones that are produced by water. For example, caffeine triggers stress responses that at first have strong diuretic effects, leading to increased urination. Beverages with added sugar raise the blood sugar level, which coerces the body to give up large quantities of water.

Other detrimental effects of some of these common beverages will be discussed in greater detail later in this book.

Chapter 3

Kidney Stones

The kidneys truly are the body's "master chemists." They not only remove waste products and excess fluids from the body via the urine, but also maintain a critical balance of salt, potassium and acid. The main responsibility of the kidneys is to keep the blood pure and healthy, and maintain proper fluid balance within the body (see **Figure 1**).

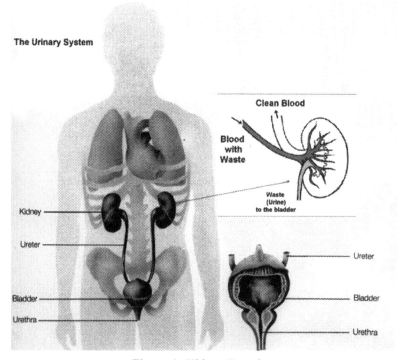

Figure 1: Kidney Functions

12

To accomplish this, the kidneys need to constantly monitor normal blood volume and filter out the right quantity of urine in order to keep it balanced. There are many factors that can disrupt this process and cause congestion in the kidneys. These factors include improper diet, dehydration, fatigue, overeating, gallstones, blood pressure disturbance, digestive disorders (especially constipation), medical or narcotic drugs, and vitamin supplements (see more on these subjects in later chapters). When the kidneys are unable to separate the necessary amounts of urine from the blood, part of the urine keeps circulating around the body, thereby depositing urinary waste products in the blood vessels, joints, tissues and organs.

Tiny crystals are formed in the kidneys when urinary constituents, which are normally in solution, are precipitated. Precipitation occurs when these particles occur in excessive amounts or when urine becomes too concentrated. Stones in the kidneys start off as tiny crystals and can eventually become as large as an egg. The tiny crystals are too small to be detected by X-rays, and since they usually do not cause pain, they are rarely noticed. Yet they are big enough to block the flow of liquid through the tiny kidney tubules. In addition, the crystal particles usually have sharp edges. Once released by the kidneys along with urine, they may cut and wear away the inner surface of the urinary canal during their passage to the urinary bladder. This can cause severe pain in the loins or lower back. There may even be blood in the urine, pain running down the legs, numbness in the thighs or difficulty in passing urine.

Most crystals or stones originate in the kidneys, although some may also be formed in the bladder. If a large stone enters one of the two urinary canals, urinary discharge becomes obstructed. This can lead to serious complications, such as kidney infection or kidney failure. Regardless of where the blockage occurs, anytime the kidneys are prevented from removing and regulating water and chemicals, these delicate organs are likely to suffer injury. The kidneys' various functions may be affected separately, so urine output may be normal despite considerable kidney disease.

Typical symptoms of congestion in the kidneys are strong body odor, water retention, abdominal swelling, rapid weight gain, high blood pressure, energy depletion, sweating of palms and feet, skin disorders, puffy eyelids and dark circles under the eyes.

Kidney Cleanse

There are various herbs that can effectively and painlessly dissolve kidney stones within a period of 3 to 6 weeks. Regardless of whether or not someone has been diagnosed with kidney stones, doing a kidney cleanse once or twice a year has tremendous curative and preventive benefits. The kidney cleanse not only improves overall physical health, but also tends to reduce stress, fear and anxieties.

Appendix B contains information about the various herbs that are effective for dissolving kidney stones and crystals. In addition, related guidelines are provided for properly administering a safe, easy and effective kidney cleanse. The book, *The Amazing Liver and Gallbladder Flush*, also contains information and guidelines for kidney cleanses.

Chapter 4

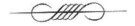

Congested Intestinal Tract

The body's health and vitality largely depend on the effortless and complete elimination of waste products from the intestinal tract. Most physical problems are caused by a build-up of waste material that may at first accumulate in the large intestine, commonly referred to as the colon, and then spread to other parts of the body, such as the liver, kidneys, heart and lungs.

When you eat highly processed foods that have been stripped of most nutrients, natural fiber and life force, the muscles wrapped around the colon have great difficulty moving along the partially digested food mass. When this substance remains in the colon for too long, it becomes progressively harder and drier. Accumulated or trapped waste material in the colon may consist of impacted feces, hardened mucus, dead cellular tissue, bacteria, parasites and various other toxic substances. Such toxins can find their way into the blood stream and lymph system, causing one to feel tired, sluggish or ill. Other common colon-related complaints include constipation, diarrhea, bloating, headaches, dizziness, nausea, sinusitis, eye and ear disorders, backaches, bad breath, body odor and disorders of the nervous system. Chronic situations are a common cause of colon cancer.

A healthy colon absorbs water, minerals and other nutrients. However, when the membrane of the colon is impacted with plaque, it cannot properly assimilate and absorb these minerals and nutrients. Accordingly, the body will begin to suffer from nutrient deficiencies. Most diseases are, in fact, deficiency disorders. They arise when certain parts of the body suffer mal-nourishment, particularly minerals. The most common cause of mal-nourishment is intestinal congestion. Stated simply, a clean colon is a prerequisite for a healthy body.

Colon Hydrotherapy

Colon hydrotherapy, also called "colonic irrigation" or simply "colonic," is perhaps one of the most effective colon therapies. Within a short period, a colonic can eliminate large amounts of trapped waste that may have taken many years to accumulate. During a 40-50 minute session of colonic hydrotherapy, a total of 2-6 liters of distilled water is used to gently flush the colon. Through gentle abdominal massage during the colonic, old deposits of hardened mucus and fecal matter are loosened and subsequently flushed out by the water.

A colonic removes not only harmful, toxic waste, but it also tones, hydrates and rejuvenates the colon muscles. The repeated uptake and release of water improves the colon's peristaltic action and reduces the transit time of fecal matter. In addition, colonic irrigation helps restore the colon's natural shape, and stimulates the reflex points that connect the colon with all the parts of the body. This form of colon cleansing can detach old crusted layers of waste from the colon walls, which permits better water absorption and hydration of the colon and the body as a whole. However, it may take at least 2-3 colonic sessions for these latter benefits to take effect.

During a colonic, one may feel a slight discomfort from time to time when larger quantities of toxic waste detach themselves from the intestinal walls and move towards the rectum. However, the feeling of lightness, cleanness and clarity of mind soon afterwards more than compensates for any feelings of mild discomfort.

Colonic irrigation can also help with emotional problems. It is no coincidence that the transverse colon passes right through the solar plexus, which is the body's emotional center. Most of our unresolved or "undigested" emotional issues are stored in the solar plexus and result in the tightening of the colon muscle. This may slow bowel movement and cause constipation. Colonics can help clear the physical obstruction and release the tension that caused the emotional repression in the first place.

Colonic cleansing is best done when the stomach is empty, or at least 2-3 hours after eating. It is beneficial to drink 1-2 glasses of water afterwards and eat a piece of fruit, or have some freshly prepared fruit juice one-half hour later. The first meal or two after the treatment should be light. After a colonic, the bowel movement will become naturally restored within about two days. If it takes longer than that, it indicates that the colon had accumulated unduly large amounts of waste over a period of many years. In this case, more colonics are recommended to remove the rest of the accumulated waste matter.

There are several different types of colon hydrotherapy systems currently in use, but all serve the same function. Professional colonic therapists receive their training from a variety of sources, but there are not yet universal standards or licensing arrangements. Fees for a colon hydrotherapy session vary considerably, but a typical one-hour session is in the range of $50 to $75.

Colema Board®

If you do not have access to a colon therapist, you may greatly benefit from using a Colema Board as a second-best choice. The Colema treatment is based on the same principle as colon-hydrotherapy, although it may not be as effective and thorough. The advantage is that the Colema Board allows you to clean your colon in the comfort of your own home. The Colema colon cleanse is a do-it-yourself treatment that is easy to learn and perform. The "Sources" page in the back of this book provides information on how to obtain a Colema Board.

Part 2

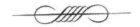

Healthy Nutrition

In the previous section, our focus was on how to keep our internal organs and systems clean, well hydrated and functioning in a healthy manner. Now it is time to discuss how to provide our body with the nutrients it needs to support a life of health and vitality.

Healthy nutrition involves a return to the simple gifts of nature – the fresh vegetables, delicious fruits, tasty seeds and nuts. Once we move beyond the fresh produce section of our local grocery store or supermarket, we can save ourselves a lot of money, and our body a lot of distress, if we leave most of the food items on the shelf, rather than putting them into our shopping cart.

Habits do not change easily. Unfortunately, the vast majority of our food preparation and eating habits in the western world are unhealthy – some dangerously so. It is human nature to assume that food producers would not market food products that are hazardous to our health. And even if some food producers and equipment manufacturers are a bit unscrupulous, we still have government "watchdog" agencies who are looking out for our best interests, don't we? In truth, such is *not* the case.

The first step in moving toward healthier nutrition is to become better informed. That is the intent of this book. From that point on, it is up to each individual to make wise choices for himself/herself, and to help make the best choices for their family – especially the children.

We wish you well!

Chapter 5

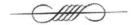

Natural Foods vs. Processed Foods

A healthy diet is one that consists primarily of "natural" foods, including vegetables, herbs, fruits, berries, grains, seeds and nuts. Unfortunately, the diet of the majority of people in the western world consists predominately of "processed" foods. Typical problems with various processed foods are:

- They are infused with harmful preservatives in order to promote "shelf life." When a food's shelf life is artificially prolonged, it does not only resist bacteria but also being digested properly.
- They tend to be laden with unhealthy sugars, sweeteners and salts, designed to appeal to our taste buds, but which are detrimental to our body.
- Many processed foods contain artificial vitamins and inorganic minerals intended to convince consumers that the food products are "enriched" in nutritional value. In reality, these synthetic vitamins and metallic minerals cannot be assimilated into the bloodstream, and only tend to clog the digestive tract and damage the kidneys and blood vessels.
- Meat and meat products are usually derived from animals that have been fed large quantities of antibiotics, growth hormones and other toxic additives, all designed to maximize production on "factory farms." The residuals of such additives find their way into the tissue of the animals and are passed onto consumers. In addition, many meat products are contaminated with illness-producing bacteria, such as Salmonella or E. coli.

19

- Some food products are "irradiated" in order to kill bacteria and promote shelf life, resulting in food that is lifeless and lacking in nutritional value. (See Chapter 18 for information of food irradiation.)
- Most processed foods contain artificial coloring and flavoring designed to appeal to the aesthetics and taste buds of the consumer, but which are toxic to the body in many cases.
- Processed foods are frequently prepared by cooking them in oil that contains significant quantities of polyunsaturated fats, resulting in food that damages or destroys cell membranes throughout the body.
- Numerous types of processed foods, such as the traditional "TV dinners," are prepared and packaged in such a way as to be conveniently heated in a microwave oven prior to eating. Microwave cooking destroys enzymes and other important nutrients, leaving essentially "dead" food that has very little nutritional value. (See Chapter 17 for information on microwave ovens.)

A diet that relies heavily on processed foods is sometimes referred to as the Standard American Diet, or "SAD" – the acronym says it all!

On the other hand, natural foods, if they are grown and prepared properly, and eaten when they are fresh, tend to provide the nutrients and life forces that are needed for a healthy body.

Modern commercial agricultural practices, unfortunately, tend to work against the production of healthy, natural foods. There has been an over-reliance on the use of chemical fertilizers that are used to increase food production. With repeated growing cycles year after year, the soil tends to be leached of its natural minerals and other life-supporting nutrients. Such agricultural practices tend to diminish the life force and nutritional value of the fruits and vegetables.

Nature has its own way of dealing with the death of plants and animals, keeping our planet tidy. When the life force diminishes, various types of microbes, fungi, insects and other "scavengers" are naturally attracted to the dying plant or animal as a source of "food." The residuals of this process then become "fertilizer" for the next generation. The concept of composting is based on this principle.

When plants are grown in leached and lifeless soil, their natural life force is diminished. Consequently, they tend to attract microbes, fungi, insects and other scavengers as part of the natural scheme of life and death. To protect the plants from such an invasion, chemical insecticides and fungicides are applied to them.

Chemicals that are used in such fertilization and protective practices tend to find their way into the fibers of the resulting vegetables, fruits and other agricultural products. Virtually all such chemicals are toxic to the human body, some more than others.

The emergence of "organic" farming is an effort to move back to more natural agricultural methods that do not rely on chemicals. Originally, "natural" food stores were the most common source of organic food products. Now that consumer awareness has heightened, organic fruits and vegetables are being sold in "specialty" sections of produce department in most mainstream supermarkets.

Since the marketing of organic produce is still in its relative infancy, uniform standards for specifying the conditions under which produce can legally be labeled as "organic" are not yet well established. So one cannot yet be absolutely certain when purchasing produce that is labeled "organic" that it is, indeed, totally chemical free. On the other hand, one can be relatively certain that produce that is not labeled "organic" probably has been subjected to at least some degree of chemical contamination.

The best possible solution to this situation is to have an organic garden of your own. In addition to being certain that the produce is raised in a chemical-free environment, there are other advantages. For example, fruits and vegetables can be eaten at their exact peak of ripeness and maturity, yielding the maximum nutritional value and tastiness. In contrast, commercial fruits and vegetables that must be harvested prior to peak maturity in order to allow for processing and distribution delays. This is a particularly important issue related to fruit, which is much healthier if eaten when it is naturally ripened. Also, for a variety of reasons related to the life force and cycles of the planet, fruits, vegetables and other natural foods are of the greatest nutritional value if they are grown in the same geographic vicinity as the area in which one lives.

Having your own organic garden is obviously much more of a challenge for city dwellers than for people who live in suburban or rural areas. In this regard, European cities have generally been much more progressive than American cities in creating "community" gardens where residents can rent a small plot in which to have their own garden or natural oasis.

Perhaps the most efficient system of growing pesticide-free fruits and vegetables is known as Sonic-Bloom (www.sonicbloom.com). The produce contains more nutrients, grows much faster and bigger and is resistant to bugs.

Chapter 6

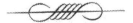

Acid-Alkaline Balance

Probably the most important factor to consider in planning healthy and nutritious meals is the acid-alkaline balance in our body.[2] The greatest cause of disease in the world today is an excess of acid-causing foods in our diet that end up as acidic residues in the cells and tissue. Cancer cells and other degenerative diseases cannot thrive in an environment that is not acidic. Even the common cold virus has difficulty surviving in an alkaline environment. Appendix D includes a list of common aliments that are frequently the result excessive acidic residues in the cells and tissues of our body.

Whether a substance is alkaline or acidic is determined by its pH (potential Hydrogen). This is a measure of the number of negative ions, which are alkaline-forming, as opposed to the number of positive ions, which are acid-forming. The standard pH scale goes from 1 to 14, with 7 being the neutral point. A substance with a pH of less than 7 is acidic, whereas one with a pH of greater than 7 is alkaline. From an energetic perspective, pH measures how much the negative ions and positive ions push against each other.

Translating this to the biochemical processes that take place within our body:

- An alkaline-forming reaction refers to any chemical alteration in the body that produces an *increased* ability to energize the system, and leaves an alkaline residue.

- An acid-forming reaction refers to any chemical alteration in the body that produces a *decreased* ability to energize the system, and leaves an acid residue.

Relating this to our food intake, natural foods such as fruits and vegetables are predominately alkaline-forming as they go through the digestive process. On the other hand, most animal proteins, processed foods and beverages are acid-forming.

If a meal has a perfect balance of alkaline-forming and acid-forming foods, then the alkaline and acids neutralize each other, and the residues will also be pH neutral. One of the problems, however, is that most fruits and vegetables are only moderately alkaline-forming, whereas many of the meat products, processed foods and beverages are extremely acid-forming. So maintaining a balance within our body is not just a matter of the *quantity* of alkaline-forming food we eat compared to acid-forming food, but also the *degree* to which the food is alkaline-forming or acid-forming.

In a healthy body, nature maintains a reserve of alkaline elements, much like a bank account. Under such circumstances, if we eat a meal that is more acidic than alkaline, our digestive processes automatically draw on the reserve of alkaline substances in our body to neutralize the acid-forming foods. But if we regularly eat meals that are overly acid-forming, the alkaline reserve in our body becomes depleted, and our body is unable to neutralize the acids. This is analogous to continuing to write checks off of a bank account without making adequate deposits – the account soon becomes overdrawn.

The 80/20 Rule

In order to assure that we regularly replenish and sustain our alkaline reserve, the best guideline to follow is the "80/20 Rule." This simply means that 80% of the foods we eat should be alkaline-forming, and 20% acid-forming. This rule does not give us license to eat acid-forming foods that may be laden with toxins such as preservatives, artificial sweeteners and other unhealthy additives. But there are certain natural foods, such as cranberries and blueberries, that although acid-forming, can be helpful in keeping our kidneys and bladder clean.

Hydrochloric Acid (HCL)

At this point, a note of clarification may be appropriate. A healthy body produces hydrochloric acid (HCL) that is essential to the digestive process. It is the only acid that our body produces. All other acids are by-products of metabolism, and are eliminated as soon as possible. HCL is the first substance in the stomach that breaks down food so that it can be metabolized. It is also our first line of defense against various destructive microbes that enter the body by way of the food we eat. HCL keeps us alive by helping to maintain a proper alkaline-acid balance, and then it becomes alkaline *after* its vital job in the digestive process is done.

List of Alkaline-forming and Acid-forming Foods

Appendix C provides a list of common foods and beverages, showing the degree to which they are alkaline-forming or acid-forming.[2][21] Fruits and vegetables are categorized based on their natural state. Any process such as cooking, freezing, canning or preserving with sugars and chemicals greatly reduces the alkaline-forming qualities – in many cases transforming them into acid-forming foods.

Ionized Water

An increasing number of counter-top water ionizers[23] are becoming readily available. Original interest in them first developed in Japan and later in South Korea. Through research by medical doctors in Japan, much valuable data has been collected. It was concluded that alkaline water made by water ionizers was non-toxic and alleviated many of the symptoms of adult diseases.

Korean-made household water ionizers were first introduced in the United States in 1985. A year later, tests were conducted by an independent laboratory using methods specified by the FDA, and no toxicity was found in alkaline water generated by the water ionizer units.

Most units incorporate a filtering process and create ionized alkaline drinking water with a pH of about 9. More time and experience will be needed to determine the long-range health benefits of this enhanced water.

Chapter 7

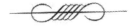

Guidelines for Healthy Meals

The previous chapter provided a perspective on *what* foods to eat. This chapter will provide some guidelines on *how* and *when* to eat them.

Cultural habits are hard to break. Dining typically involves not only the consumption of food and beverages, but also provides an opportunity for social interaction. Unfortunately, the eating habits of most people in the western world are detrimental to the promotion of health and vitality.

There are several factors that need to be taken into consideration. First and most importantly, each of us has a unique body, with unique nutritional requirements. One person may thrive on a particular food that might make another person ill. Or, foods that support our health in the winter months may not agree with us in the summer months. And, a food that may be nurturing to our health if eaten at midday may be detrimental to our health if eaten in the evening. The ancient science of *Ayurveda*, as discussed in Chapter 8, addresses a wide range of variables, and provides guidelines for several different body types. However, there are some general "rules of thumb" that apply to most of us, based on the manner in which our bodies process food. Let's start with the question of raw versus cooked natural foods.

Raw versus Cooked

Since heating foods kills enzymes and alters other nutrients, it would seem that eating a diet of nothing but raw natural food, such as fruits and vegetables, would be ideal. There certainly are a lot of other mammals that live on such a diet, and they seem to do just fine. And with the growth of raw food diets and menus catering to them, it appears that raw foods' popularity is increasing. But it is not quite that simple.

Our digestive tracts need fiber in order properly process the foods we eat. Fiber is the "skeleton" of plants. Its primary role in our digestive process is to stimulate waves of muscular contractions which move the food along through the intestines. There is a commonly held belief that fiber cannot be digested, and leaves our body unaltered. But this applies only to the small intestine. In the large intestine (colon), fiber is attacked and broken down by a large number of "residential" bacteria. This can result in fermentation if the fiber does not pass through the colon in a reasonable amount of time.

Cooked vegetables and grains contain fiber which helps the digestive process, but does not overwhelm the colon. Also, the high water content of cooked foods generally makes the passage through the intestinal tract much easier. While raw fresh vegetables contain the same fiber as cooked foods, it requires more time and energy to process raw foods through the intestines. Certain body types are more capable of dealing with large quantities of raw food. Many people have gone on virtually 100% raw food diets and have thrived on such a diet for extended periods of time. But in some cases, after as long as 10 or 20 years, their bodies began to suffer a physical breakdown. They could no longer cope with the breaking down of hard grains and raw vegetables.

The fiber in fruits is also beneficial to the digestive process. But ripened fruits have already been "cooked" by the sun. So cooking by artificial means is not necessary.

The safest approach is to maintain a reasonable balance between raw and cooked foods in our daily diet. If adjustments are made to increase the proportion of raw food, they should be made gradually so that the body is able to accommodate it accordingly.

The inclusion of raw vegetable juices in a person's diet helps to provide enzymes and nutrients to offset those that are altered in the cooking process. Also, sprouting grains and seeds, as discussed in Chapter 9, is a good compliment to cooking.

If raw foods and cooked foods are combined in the same meal, raw foods, such as salads or fresh vegetable juice, should always be eaten first.

Food Combining

Each type of food is processed through the digestive tract in a different manner, and requires different types of enzymes and other digestive agents.[20] Additionally, certain foods move through the digestive tract much more quickly than others.

A list of the most common foods in each food group is shown in Appendix E. An explanatory note may be helpful here. In the chapter on acid-alkaline balance, it was indicated that most fruits are alkaline-forming. Yet, in the list of foods in Appendix E, certain fruits are listed as acidic, or sub-acidic in nature. Although this may seem like a contradiction, it is not. For example, we know that oranges contain citric acid. But as oranges are metabolized in the body, certain minerals are *acid-binding*. This means that in the body, they *bind* acid toxins, leaving a residual that is *alkaline*. So, from the perspective of how acidic fruits impact the body after digestion, they are alkaline-forming.

Following are guidelines for combining, or not combining, foods from the various food groups in the same meal.

Proteins and Starches

Do not combine proteins and starches – this is the worst possible combination to mix together in a single meal, even though it is the mainstay of most western meals. Protein food requires an acid medium for digestion, whereas starch foods require an alkaline medium for proper digestion. When one consumes protein and starch together, the alkaline enzyme ptyalin pours into the food as it is chewed in the mouth. When the masticated food reaches the stomach, digestion of starch by alkaline enzymes continues unabated, thereby preventing the digestion of protein by pepsin and other acid secretions. As a result, the ever-present bacteria in the stomach are permitted to attack the protein, and putrefaction commences, rendering nutrients in the protein food largely useless, and producing toxic waste and foul gases.

Proteins and Fruits

Proteins should not be eaten along with fruits – especially not acid fruits. This may seem counter-intuitive, since proteins require an acid environment in order to be digested. However, when acid foods enter the stomach, they inhibit the secretion of hydrochloric acid. The protein-digesting enzyme, *pepsin*, can work only in the presence of hydrochloric acid, not just any acid. Also, fruits pass through the digestive tract much more quickly than proteins. If eaten in the same meal, the protein foods delay the movement of fruits through the stomach and intestines, causing fermentation.

Proteins and Green Vegetables

Protein foods combine well with green vegetables. However, if the green vegetables are raw, such as in a salad, they should be eaten prior to the protein food.

Proteins and Proteins

In general, it is best to include only one protein food in a meal, since different types of protein foods are processed differently. For example, the strongest enzymatic action on meat occurs in the first hour of digestion, whereas on cheese, it occurs during the last hour. However, it is not a serious problem to combine similar protein foods.

Fruits and Starches

Fresh ripened fruits undergo little or no digestion in the mouth and stomach. They move quickly into the small intestine where they undergo the little digestion they require. If fruit is eaten with a different type of food, such as a piece of bread (starch), the fruit is held up in the stomach along with the bread until the bread is ready to move on to the intestines. This delay causes the fruit to begin to ferment in the stomach. The by-products of fermentation are acidic, which further inhibit digestion of the bread, a starch that requires an alkaline medium for digestion. Additionally, when a piece of bread is eaten by itself, the saliva glands in the mouth secrete ptyalin, a digestive agent that is needed by the bread for proper digestion. But if fruit is eaten along with the bread, the natural sugars in the fruit block the secretion of ptyalin, further complicating digestion of the bread.

Fruits and Green Vegetables

Fruits generally do not combine well with green vegetables. However, vegetables such as carrots can be eaten with most fruit.

Fruits and Fruits

Various types of sweet fruits can be combined with each other, but should not be combined with acid fruits. Sub-acid fruits are half way in between, and can be combined with either sweet fruits or acid fruits, but not both. See Appendix E for a list of fruits in the various categories.

Melons

The general rule is that melons should be eaten alone. They require no digestion in the stomach, and pass quickly through the intestines for digestion and assimilation. If combined with anything, melons should only be taken with fresh raw fruits. But it is best to eat them alone.

Other Guidelines for Meals

- The main meal of the day should be eaten at mid-day when the sun is at its apex and digestive powers are the strongest, rather than in the evening when digestive strength is greatly subdued. And foods should not be eaten just before going to bed. There should be at least 3 hours between the last meal of the day and bedtime. Otherwise, food may remain undigested in the stomach, causing fermentation, bloating or discomfort, and even weight gain.
- Avoid drinking beverages with a meal, since this dilutes the body's concentrated digestive juices, resulting in indigestion and weight gain. It is especially important not to use beverages to "wash the food down" prematurely into the stomach. If you desire to drink anything during a meal, it is best to sip warm water or perhaps a mild herbal tea.
- Chew foods well – especially meat and other hard-to-digest foods. Chewing is an important part of the digestive process.
- Keep meals simple – generally no more than 3 or 4 different foods.
- Raw foods should be eaten before cooked foods.
- Eat juicy foods prior to concentrated, solid foods.
- Eat more raw foods in summer, less in winter.
- Eat foods and beverages at room temperature, or warmer if cooked.
- With the exception of beans and rice, it is not advisable to retain "leftovers" for meals the following day, because they have no life force left in them after a few hours.

- Meals should be eaten in a peaceful environment, with only pleasant company. It is best not to eat while the mind is dominated by strong emotions such as fear or anger.
- Do not over-indulge at mealtime. As the internal organs of the body are cleansed and revitalized, and as we eliminate toxic "junk" foods from our diet, our digestive processes become much more efficient. Consequently, we can gain all of the nutrients our body needs with less total food intake.
- Ayurveda teaches that we should include a balance of all six taste types in our daily meals: sweet, sour, salty, pungent, bitter and astringent. However, certain body types may have a predisposition for one taste over another.
- Avoid sleeping right after a meal, as that can cause sluggishness and weight gain. An ideal situation is to rest for 10-15 minutes after a meal and then go for a 10-15 minute walk.

Chapter 8

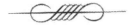

Ayurveda

A Natural Approach to Health and Well-Being

Ayurveda, which translates to "science of longevity," has its origins in the culture of ancient India. The primary focus of Ayurvedic Medicine is on maintaining a balanced relationship with the world in which we live.

According to Ayurveda, everything in the universe is made up of combinations of five elements. These five elements are to be understood in a material sense as well as a subtle sense:

- **Space** (Akasha): This is the most subtle of the 5 elements; it is everywhere and touches everything. In the mind, it is the vessel that receives all impressions; in the heart it accepts love. Space is receptivity and non-resistance to what is true.
- **Air** (Vayu): This is the transparent, rarefied, kinetic force that sets the universe in motion. Air moves the blood through the vessels, wastes from the body, and thoughts through the mind. It also moves the birds to warmer climates in winter, and moves the planets around their suns.
- **Fire** (Tejas): Fire is the universal force in nature that produces heat and radiates light. It is our passion to pursue despite obstacles and delays; it is what burns away the cloak of ignorance and allows the truth to shine with brilliance. Fire removes doubt from the mother-substance of the human heart and replaces it with joy.
- **Water** (Apa): Water comprises the cohesive aspects of reality that flow into and hold things together – perfectly

and simply witnessed in the ubiquitous H_2O molecule. The other elements were also intended by the ancients to communicate the essential universal principle inherent in a particular element.

- **Earth** (Prithvi): This is the terrain of our planet, the iron in our red blood cells and spleen. It also represents the quality of steadfastness of mind, strength of moral fiber, one's slow and quiet undeterred advancement towards a goal, and the resistance to the actions of others.

The five elements can be seen to exist within all aspects of the material universe. When they enter into the biology of a living organism, such as a human being, they acquire a biological form. This means that the five elements are coded into three biological forces which govern all life processes. These three forces are known as the three *doshas*. The three doshas regulate every physiological and psychological process in the living organism. The interplay among them determines the qualities and conditions of the individual. A harmonious state of the three doshas creates balance and health. An imbalance, which might be an excess or deficiency, manifests as a sign or symptom of disease. Following is a brief description of each of the doshas:

- **Vata** (Space and Air): The term vata means "that which moves things." It is composed of the elements space and air – the lightest and subtlest of the five elements. It is considered in some ways to be the most influential of the three doshas because it is the moving force behind the other two. Vata is responsible for all movements in the mind and body: the movement of air in and out of the lungs, the flow of blood through the circulatory system, nutrients through the alimentary tract, and thoughts through the mind. Vata promotes a healthy balance between thought and emotion, and gives rise to creativity, activity and clear comprehension.

- **Pitta** (Fire and Water): Pitta is often regarded as the "fire" within the body. One may think of it as the energy stored in the chemical bonds of all the organic substances which make up our body. It is encoded in our hormones, enzymes, organic acids and neurotransmitters. Pitta also carries the meaning of "that which digests" and is associated with the body's digestive function, including all chemical and metabolic transformations, and processes that promote heat. Pitta governs our ability to digest ideas and impressions, and to therefore perceive the true nature of reality.

- **Kapha** (Water and Earth): The term kapha means "that which holds things together." It is the force that provides structure to everything, from an individual atom or cell, to the sturdy musculoskeletal frame. It gives strength, stability and endurance – both physical and psychological – and promotes human emotions and capacities such as love, compassion, empathy, understanding, forgiveness, loyalty and patience. One very important function of kapha in the human body is governing immunity and resistance against disease. Its energy promotes self-healing and the ongoing processes of self-repair, of which we are largely unaware. Whereas the effects of vata and pitta become active in the body, Kapha acts to limit and control these two forces, and prevent their excessive activity.

One may think of these doshas as fundamental biological energies that regulate all the life processes of an individual. All three doshas function within each of us. However, we each have them in unique proportions. Consequently, one person might be predominately a vata type person, with lesser aspects of pitta or kapha. Or, another person might be primarily kapha, with lesser influence from vata or pitta.

Figure 1 illustrates the relationship between the elements and doshas. As may be noted, each of the three doshas is shown at each of the three corners of the triangle, along with the two elements to which each dosha is related. Each one of us could find our unique place on the triangular chart. If we had a perfect balance of all three doshas, we would be in the exact center of the triangle. However, a perfect balance would be very unusual. If we were predominately vata in nature, our position on the chart would be toward the upper apex of the triangle.

Ayurveda: The Elements and Doshas

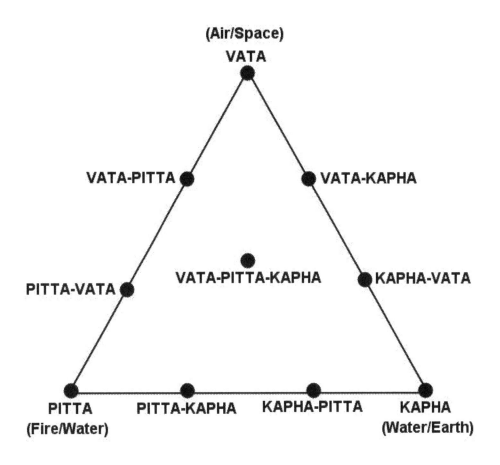

Figure 1: The dosha pyramid

For the purpose of simplification, Ayurvedic health practices deal with 10 different basic body types. Each is illustrated by one of the black dots on the diagram.

Ayurvedic Nutrition

Since every living plant also consists of the 5 elements, every vegetable, fruit, herb, seed, nut and so on has qualities related to the three doshas. As indicated earlier, the primary focus of Ayurveda is on maintaining the appropriate balance in relationship to the universe in which we live. This includes a consideration of natural cycles such as the four seasons, the moon phases and, of course, the daily cycles of night and day. In light of this, dietary planning for each individual takes into account the natural cycles as well as which of the 10 basic body types most closely matches the person's unique nature.

The book, *Timeless Secrets of Health and Rejuvenation*, provides detailed information on how to determine your own unique body type, and also includes comprehensive meal planning and health enhancing guidelines for each of the basic body types.

Chapter 9

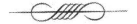

Sprouts

Seeds are rich in nutrients. After all, they contain all of the nutrients that are necessary to create the initial shoot of a growing plant. Nevertheless, it is difficult for the human body to fully digest and assimilate the nutrients that are present within most seeds.

A good solution to this dilemma is to enable the seeds to germinate and sprout into small shoots. Such sprouts are much easier for the body to assimilate. And the process of sprouting alters the chemistry of the original seed – most notably, making it much less starchy. Also, as the seeds are exposed to sunlight in the later stages of the sprouting process, photosynthesis occurring within the plant creates significant quantities of chlorophyll, an important health enhancer. The sprouting of seeds also develops Vitamin A and Vitamin C in a form that is easily assimilated by the body.

For many years, the late Ann Wigmore generated a lot of interest around the use of wheat sprouts, or "wheatgrass," as a way to detoxify the body and improve vitality.[24] Although the conventional medical community challenged some of the claims related to wheatgrass being an anti-cancer agent and a food that enhanced longevity, literally thousands of people around the world continue to benefit from Ann's pioneering work.

Perhaps the most common seeds used for sprouting are alfalfa seeds. Alfalfa sprouts can be found in the produce section of almost any modern supermarket. Virtually any seeds can be sprouted, and it is not uncommon to use a mixture of seeds in the same sprouting container. One of the more difficult seeds to sprout is sesame. But sesame has its own magic and does not need to be sprouted in order for the body to assimilate its beneficial nutrients, such as calcium.

Sprouts are commonly eaten in salads and sandwiches. But they can also be put through a juicing machine and combined with vegetable juices. Ann Wigmore indicated that juice from wheatgrass retained its life force nutrients for no more than three hours at most. The same may be true of other types of sprout juices. Sprouts can be effectively juiced in some of the juicing machines currently on the market, such as "twin gear" type juicers. Due to the popularity of wheatgrass as a health enhancer, there are commercial juicers that have been specifically designed to juice wheat sprouts. Most of these are effective for other types of sprouts as well.

Juice from sprouts such as alfalfa, which is high in chlorophyll, is really quite potent. Consequently, it is usually best to combine sprout juices with vegetable juices such as carrot or celery juice. This also provides a "tasty" base that, at least for some people, makes sprout juices more palatable.

Another advantage of sprouts is that they can be grown in a relatively small space. So even apartment dwellers can grow sprouts and enjoy watching the miracle of nature as tiny seeds germinate and grow into little plants. Various types of seeds for growing sprouts can be found in virtually all "natural" or "health" food stores. Grains and seeds that will sprout can also be found in agricultural supply stores, but often such seeds have been treated with anti-fungal or other chemicals that are hazardous to our health. So, as a general rule, it is wise to obtain seeds and grains for sprouting only from traditional food outlets, rather than from agricultural stores. There is a wide selection of books currently available that provide guidance on how to sprout seeds.

Note: Not everyone benefits from sprouts and wheatgrass juice or other juices. For example, the vata body type may become constipated or develop intestinal gas from sprouts, and the pitta type may get irritated by the large concentration of antibodies that make up a part of the immune system in wheat grass (for the purpose of self-defense against insects and worms). Although these antibodies can trigger powerful cleansing reactions in the body, taken in large amounts or on an ongoing basis, they can weaken the body's immune system and cause gas, bloating and irritability.

Chapter 10

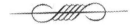

Raw Vegetable Juices

Fresh vegetables are perhaps the most important component of a healthy diet. They contain natural vitamins, minerals and other nutrients that are essential to our health and vitality. They also contain living enzymes that are required for the digestive, metabolic and assimilation processes within the digestive tract.[8]

Enzymes are sensitive to heat. At temperatures above 118° F, they start to become sluggish, just as the human body becomes lethargic in a hot bath. At temperatures above 130° F, enzymes die. A dead enzyme cannot perform its crucial role in the digestive processes of the body.

In Chapter 7, the pros and cons of cooked food versus raw foods are discussed. Raw solid food requires many hours of digestive activity before its nourishment is available to the cells and tissues of the body. Cooked foods are more easily digested. But since cooking foods kills the enzymes, we are faced with a dilemma. Converting some of our raw vegetables into juices is a good way to accommodate this situation.

In contrast to the long period of time needed to digest raw vegetables, the nutrients of vegetable juices can be absorbed into the bloodstream in a matter of minutes, rather than hours. And the process of juicing, using any of a wide variety of kitchen juicers currently on the market, does not damage or compromise the enzymes or other nutrients in the vegetables.[22]

There is another advantage that raw vegetable juices have over solid vegetables. Residuals of chemical fertilizers and pesticides that are assimilated into the vegetables reside primarily in the fiber of the vegetables. Since the fiber of the vegetables becomes a waste product in the juicing process, raw vegetable juices provide a way to derive the nutritious benefit of vegetables without ingesting harmful residual chemicals.

A certain amount of fiber is important to the digestive process, since it acts as a "broom" to help keep the intestinal tract clean. Consequently it is important to continue to include solid vegetables, cooked and uncooked, as a staple in our daily diet. Vegetable juices tend to consist of highly concentrated nutrients, so they should be introduced into our daily diet with appropriate caution.

There is yet another virtue of raw vegetable juices. Chapter 6 discusses the importance of maintaining an appropriate acid/alkaline balance in the body. Most foods and beverages tend toward being acidic. However, most vegetables are alkaline. By drinking raw vegetable juices, we not only help bring about the necessary hydration of the body, but we also help to alkalize the body.

If there is a downside to raw vegetable juices, it is probably the fact that the nutrients in the juice begin to break down fairly soon after the juicing process – in a matter of hours, rather than days. Consequently, it is important to drink vegetable juices reasonably soon after the juicing process. In busy households, in which time and convenience are at a premium, this can present a challenge.

To some extent, the effective "shelf life" of raw vegetable juice depends on the juicing process that is used. As previously indicated, there are a wide variety of kitchen juicers currently on the market:

- Perhaps the most common types are *centrifugal* juicers that spin at a very high speed. These work quite well for rigid vegetables such as carrots or celery, but they do not work well, if at all, for leafy vegetables, sprouts or herbs. Another disadvantage is that the grinding friction resulting from the high-speed rotation tends to create a certain amount of heat – not enough to damage the enzymes, but enough to shorten the shelf life of the juice.

- Another type of juicer is a *masticating* juicer. These produce a vegetable juice with a slightly longer shelf life than centrifugal juicers – in the range of 24 hours.

- A third type is known as a *twin-gear* juicer. These work well for most types of vegetables, including leafy vegetables, herbs and sprouts. And they produce a juice with a slightly longer shelf life. However, it is always best to drink vegetable and fruit juice within an hour after making it.
- There are also various *specialty* juicers, such as those specifically designed for wheatgrass.

Most vegetable juicers can also be used for certain types of fruits. Fruit juices require special consideration, since they tend to have a high natural sugar content.

To understand which types of vegetable juices are most beneficial, one needs to do a bit of research into the nutritional value of the vegetables from which they are derived. Chapter 16, entitled, "Foods with Special Health Enhancing Qualities", provides some clues. Following are a few of the more common vegetable juices, along with their primary attributes:

- **Carrot juice**: A rich source of Vitamin A, and also contains Vitamins B, C, D, E, G and K. It is very beneficial for nursing mothers, as it helps insure that the breast milk will contain important vitamins and nutrients. It also aids overall digestion. Because it is quite flavorful, it is a good juice to mix with other vegetable juices that are less appealing to the palate.
- **Celery juice**: Contains a high quantity of vital organic sodium. Organic sodium is important in its role of maintaining calcium in solution so that it can be assimilated where needed throughout the body.
- **Alfalfa juice**: Is rich in minerals and trace elements because of the deep root system of the alfalfa plant. Also

rich in chlorophyll, which is derived from the rays of the sun. Chlorophyll enhances the vital life energy of the body.[10]

- **Beet juice**: One of the most valuable juices for building up the red corpuscles of the blood. Because it also has a cleansing effect on the liver, it is best not to drink more than one-third of a cup of pure beet juice per day, otherwise it can cause a toxic reaction. It is best to start the use of beet juice by mixing small quantities of it with carrot juice.
- **Cucumber juice**: Is high in potassium, and is a natural diuretic – secreting and promoting the flow of urine. It also promotes hair growth due to a high content of silicon.
- **Parsley juice**: Is one of the most potent juices, and should never be taken in quantities of more than 1 or 2 ounces at a time. It is best to mix it with other juices, such as carrot or celery juice. It facilitates oxygen metabolism and also helps maintain normal functioning of the adrenal and thyroid glands. Like alfalfa juice, parsley juice is rich in chlorophyll.[10]

As with all natural foods, certain types of vegetable juices may be beneficial for one person, but not beneficial, or even detrimental, to another. And if significant quantities of a particular juice are consumed over a period of time, the body may begin to develop an adverse reaction, even though the juice may have been beneficial in the beginning. Therefore, just as it is good to eat a variety of vegetables, it may also be beneficial to drink a variety of juices.

The best way to monitor the effects of raw vegetable juices in one's diet is to test them occasionally, using the muscle testing technique described in Appendix A.

Important note: Juices are actually only beneficial if they are "chewed" and saturated with salivary enzymes in the mouth before swallowing. Drinking juices as you would drink water will not just make their precious nutrients unavailable to the cells of your body, but may actually cause gas and bloating in the gastrointestinal tract. To digest the sugars contained in fruit and vegetable juices, they need to be combined with enzymes contained in the saliva. Otherwise, they will simply ferment and turn into low-grade alcohol that is toxic for the body.

Chapter 11

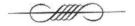

Meat

Is eating meat healthy for us, or not? That is the basic question that will be addressed in this chapter.

The *Oxford Vegetarian Study* was a 15 year research effort that began in Oxford, England in the early 1980's. A total of 11,000 volunteers participated in the study; 6,000 vegetarians and 5,000 non-vegetarians. The results of the study indicated that meat eaters are twice as likely to die from heart disease, have a 60% greater risk of dying from cancer and a 30% higher risk of death from other diseases. In fairness, vegetarians are likely to be more careful with other aspects of their dietary intake, such as processed foods that are known to be unhealthy. So the above statistics may not be totally attributable to a meat, versus non-meat diet.

The American National Institute of Health, in a study of 50,000 vegetarians, found that the vegetarians live longer and also have an impressively lower incidence of heart disease, and a significantly lower rate of cancer than meat-eating Americans.

Researcher Rollo Russell writes in his *Notes on the Causation of Cancer:* "I have found of twenty-five nations eating flesh largely, nineteen had a high cancer rate and only one had a low rate, and that of thirty-five nations eating little or no flesh, none of these had a high rate."

A major study conducted in California revealed that the cancer rate among Mormons, who are known to eat very little meat, was 50% lower than in the normal population. An even more comprehensive, 8-year controlled study on 50,000 vegetarians of the *Seventh Day Adventist* church in California, compared with the same number of non-vegetarians of the same sex and age, produced similar results as in *the Oxford Vegetarian Study*. The study, which was completed in 1966, found that members of the vegetarian group had an astonishingly low rate of cancer of all types, their life expectancy was significantly longer, and they suffered significantly less from cardiovascular disease than those in the control group.

In the same context, the "forced" vegetarianism of the Danes, due to the allied blockage of Denmark in World War I, led to a 17% reduction of mortality rates in the first year of meat rationing. Norway experienced a similar positive side effect from meat rationing during the years of World War II (1940-1945). There was an immediate drop in national mortality rates from circulatory diseases during the period of meat shortage. The rates returned to pre-war levels when the population resumed meat consumption.

In June 1961, the American Medical Association reported that a vegetarian diet could prevent 90% of our thrombo-embolic disease and 97% of our coronary occlusions. This means that by adopting a vegetarian diet, we would be able to almost completely eradicate heart disease.

There are two aspects that need to be considered related to the impact of meat on human health:

- The meat, itself, and how it is assimilated into the body.
- Additives and medications that are fed to animals on modern "factory farms," and the potential contamination of meat during its processing and distribution.

Digestion of Meat

Let's start with the meat, itself. Animal cells, unlike plant cells that have a rigid cell wall and a simple circulatory system, die very rapidly once they are cut off from their blood supply. When the animal dies, its cell proteins coagulate and destructive enzymes immediately begin to break down the cells. This, in turn, results in the formation of a degenerative substance called *ptomaine,* which is a known cause of many diseases. Cellular destruction applies to the cells of all types of dead animal flesh, as well as chicken and fish. All meat is contaminated with decomposed and putrefied protein, as well as worms and parasites that are involved in the breakdown of the protein structures. A dead animal, bird or fish is no longer "fresh" regardless what you do with it. Clever preservation methods such as refrigerating and adding carcinogenic preservatives to the meat doesn't bring it back to life or make any fresher. Putrefaction and bacterial growth start immediately after death and are very advanced by the time the meat is several days old.

Next, let's consider the digestive process. At the heart of the problem lies our inability to properly break down meat protein into amino acids. In a carnivorous animal, unlike in a human, the main digestive work takes place in the stomach, not in the small intestine. Meat stays in their relatively short intestinal tract for only a brief period of time.

In a human, however, chunks of undigested meat pass from the stomach into the intestinal tract. Our small intestine, which is about 16-20 feet (5-6 meters) long, processes most natural foods within a matter of several hours. But if the food happens to be meat, it may stay in the intestinal tract for as long as 24 to 48 hours. By that time, much of it is putrefied or decayed. The rotting process results in the generation of the meat poisons *cadaverine, putrescine* and other toxic substances.

Since the remnants of undigested meat can be held in the large intestinal walls of humans for 20-30 years or longer, it is not surprising to find colon cancers to be so highly prevalent among meat eaters, but virtually non-existent among carnivorous animals and vegetarians. Colon cancer, in most cases, is just another name for constant poisoning through putrefying meat. While being digested, meat is known to generate *steroid metabolites* possessing *carcinogenic* (cancer-producing) properties. In addition, the heating of meat at high temperatures creates chemicals that are not found in uncooked meats, including *Heterocyclic Amines (HCAs)*. These poisons begin to act as pathogens (causal factors of disease) in the body. According to research conducted by the National Cancer Institute (NCI) as well as European and Japanese researchers, there are 17 different HCAs resulting from the cooking of muscle meats, such as beef, pork, fowl, and fish, that may pose human cancer risk (for more information, see references to 21 studies on the NCI's website:

_http://www.cancer.gov/cancertopics, under the category, "factsheet/Risk/heterocyclic-amines").

The kidneys, which extract waste products from the blood, also suffer from the overload of meat poisons, consisting mostly of nitrogenous wastes. Even moderate meat eaters demand three times more work from their kidneys than do vegetarians. Generally speaking, young people may still be able to cope with this form of stress, but as they grow older the risk of kidney damage greatly increases.

After many years of regularly consuming meat, the body may suddenly succumb to the flood of poisonous substances emanating from undigested meat. A research study conducted in Germany showed that middle-aged people who consumed meat in the evening were more prone to suffer a heart attack during the next morning. Too many proteins entering the blood can thicken it and drastically cut oxygen supplies to the heart and other organs, such as the brain.

Medications and Additives

In his groundbreaking 1987 book, *Diet for a New America*, John Robbins discussed the inhumane and unhealthy ways in which animals are raised on contemporary "factory farms." One of the areas of great concern is the prolific use of additives, pesticides, hormones, growth and appetite stimulants, tranquilizers and antibiotics that are employed in the rearing of animals for meat consumption.

A 10-year study of government data that was completed in 2003 found that approximately 30 million pounds of antibiotics are used in America each year.[17] Of this amount, 25 million pounds are used in the raising of farm animals! According to a report by the

FDA, the antibiotics *penicillin* and *tetracycline* alone save the meat industry $1.9 billion a year. Yet the drugs may be breeding deadly antibiotic-resistant organisms in the consumer's body.

One of the chemicals added to animal feed in the United States is the growth hormone *diethylstilbestrol* (DES). The FDA estimates that it saves American meat producers $500 million annually. DES is highly carcinogenic and banned as a serious health hazard in 32 countries.

Unfortunately, the "farms" of an earlier era have become the "pharms" of the modern day agri-business. There are over 2,500 drugs routinely given to animals to fatten them and to keep them alive. Most of the harmful chemicals are still in the animals at the time of death, and many other drugs are added after the animal has been slaughtered. These drugs will still be present in the meat when it is eaten. Unfortunately, the law does not require listing of the vast array of drugs added to the meat.

Another reason why meat eaters have more cancers than vegetarians may be the fact that they ingest large quantities of sodium nitrates and sodium nitrites, which are carcinogenic preservatives used to make the meat look "fresh." As already mentioned, meat is no longer fresh after the animal is dead. If left untreated, animal flesh begins to turn into a sickly gray-green color within several days. Since nobody would buy the meat in that condition, the meat industry uses these toxic chemicals to camouflage the decay and make it look red and palatable, whereas in reality it is already decomposed and highly toxic. These preservatives are especially prevalent in processed meat such as salami, hot dogs, pepperoni and bologna.

Meat Contamination

Research has shown that *all* meat eaters have worms and a high incidence of parasites in the intestines. This is hardly surprising given the fact that dead flesh is a favorite target for micro-organisms of all sorts. A 1996 study by the U. S. Department of Agriculture showed that nearly 80% of ground beef is contaminated with disease-causing microbes. The primary source of these bugs is feces. A 2005 study conducted by the University of Arizona found there are more fecal bacteria in the average kitchen sink than in the average toilet bowl. The source of this biohazard at home is the meat you buy at the typical grocery store or supermarket.

The germs and parasites found in meat weaken the immune system and are the source of many diseases. In fact, most food poisonings today are related to meat eating. During a mass outbreak near Glasgow, 16 out of over 200 infected people died from the consequences of eating E. coli contaminated meat. There are occasional outbreaks reported in many other parts of the world. More than half a million Americans, most of whom are young people, have been sickened by mutant fecal bacteria (E. coli) in meat. These germs are the leading cause of kidney failure among children in the United States. Not all parasites act so swiftly as *E. coli* though. Most of them have long-term effects that are noticed only after many years of eating meat.

There are new mutant bugs found in today's meat that are extremely deadly. For you to come down with Salmonella poisoning, you would have to consume at least a million of these germs. But to become infected with one of the new mutant bugs, you would only have to ingest a measly five of them. In other words, a tiny particle of uncooked hamburger, making it from a kitchen utensil to your plate, is enough to kill you. Scientists have now identified more than a dozen food-borne pathogens with such disastrous consequences. The U. S. Center of Disease Control admits that we don't even know the bugs behind most food-related illnesses and deaths.

Fish

Many of the issues related to red meat and poultry apply to fish as well. Fish raised in commercial fish tanks are subject to much of the same chemical contamination as animals raised on "factory farms." And with the increasing pollution of our oceans, rivers and lakes, increasing levels of toxic chemicals and substances, such as mercury, are found in fish and shellfish that are harvested from the Earth's natural bodies of water.

Chapter 12

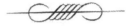

Milk

Dairy milk has become a major target of criticism over the past few years due to its long list of negative side effects. More and more health practitioners report that patients are allergic to dairy products or suffer from food intolerance to milk-containing foods. Eczema, asthma, migraine headaches, constipation, hay fever, arthritis, stomach trouble, heart disease and testicular cancer are all linked with high consumption of dairy products.

Could it be that cow's milk is meant only for calves just as cat's milk is meant only for kittens? Would we consider feeding our babies with dog's milk, for example, instead of human breast milk? The ratio of nutrients contained in dog's milk does not suit human requirements. Yet the same applies to cow's milk. Cow's milk contains three times as much protein and almost four times as much calcium as a human mother's milk. These amounts are unsuitable for the human physiology at any age.

Cow's milk is designed to contain the exact amount of calcium and protein necessary to feed a calf that will end up being at least 3-4 times larger than a human body. If we gave human breast milk to a calf, it would not grow strong enough to survive. By contrast, human babies require more carbohydrates in the beginning stages of their lives than calves do. For this reason, cow's milk contains only 50% of the carbohydrates found in human milk. Calves, on the other hand, require more salt than human babies do, so salt content in cow's milk is three times higher than in human milk. It is, therefore, not surprising that most of the indigenous populations living in Asia, Africa, Australia and South America do not regard cow's milk as a food fit for human consumption.

Once weaned, mammals no longer look for milk to satisfy their hunger or thirst. It has been speculated that if human babies who have been breast-fed for a year were given the option of choosing from various types of natural foods, most would no longer want breast milk as a food. Babies who are fed with cow's milk tend to look puffy, bloated and fat. It is not uncommon for 1-year olds to have gallstones in the liver as a result of drinking, and not digesting, cow's milk. Many of them suffer from colic and gas that makes them cry and develop sleeping problems.

Michael Klaper, M.D., author of *Vegan Nutrition: Pure & Simple*, summarized the milk controversy as follows: "The human body has no more need for cows' milk than it does for dogs' milk, horses' milk, or giraffes' milk."

Cow's milk is a highly mucus-forming food that can cause irritation and congestion throughout the gastro-intestinal tract. If regularly consumed, milk can leave an increasingly hardening and almost impermeable coating on the inside of the intestinal membranes. This restricts absorption of nutrients, including the calcium, magnesium and zinc needed to form bones. It is virtually impossible to treat people nutritionally as long as they continue to clog up their digestive systems with milk or dairy foods.

Milk-caused Osteoporosis

Most people wouldn't drink milk if they weren't so influenced by the myth that milk is essential for the bones. If you are prone to osteoporosis, or osteoarthritis, then consider the following facts:[18]

- Cow's milk may be very rich in calcium but its high calcium-to-magnesium ratio can make it difficult to absorb. In certain people or body types, calcium may be deposited in places where it is not required, hence the development of calcification of bones and other body parts. Most of the calcium contained in cow's milk is bound by the milk chemical *casein*, which makes it far too crude for proper absorption by the human intestinal membranes. Cow's milk contains 300 times more casein than human milk. You can get more absorbable calcium out of 6-8 almonds or a teaspoon of molasses than you can from one liter of cow's milk.

- There is quantitatively more phosphorus in cow's milk than there is calcium. To metabolize that much phosphorus, the body requires extra amounts of calcium, which it extracts from the bones, teeth and muscles. This leads to a calcium deficiency in these parts of the body. If the consumption of dairy foods continues for a long time, the calcium reserves get depleted faster than they can be replenished, leading to damage of the bone tissue.

- Cows maintain strong and hardy bones and teeth throughout their lives and get most of their calcium from the greens they eat. Likewise, gorillas, elephants and other strong animals do not suffer from osteoporosis. Occasionally they lick on limestone, but this is certainly not enough to supply the large quantities of calcium they require to build and rebuild their heavy skeletons. If milk were the most useful and important source of calcium for grown animals, then nature would certainly have designed ways of supplying them with milk throughout their lives. But as we know, they have access to milk only at the beginning stages of their lives.

Acid-Alkaline Balance

Milk proteins contain about three times as many sulfur-containing amino acids as vegetable proteins. Through regular consumption of milk and dairy products, the blood would become too acidic if the body did not mobilize large amounts of minerals to save the body from acid death. In the long term, this emergency measure leads to demineralization of the tissues and organs, and eventually acidosis.

Low Fat Milk

To digest whole milk, the human body requires large amounts of bile. Regularly drinking whole milk can eventually exhaust the liver's bile-producing capacity. Switching to low fat milk makes matters even worse. Although low fat milk requires less bile to digest the fat contained in the milk, milk protein cannot be digested without the natural amounts of milk fat. Large amounts of undigested milk protein increase acidity in the body, and the unused crude milk calcium can cause calcification of joints, arteries or kidneys.

Allergies

Whey is a liquid by-product of the production of cheese. It has been touted by the food industry as containing important health nutrients. Since nobody really likes drinking this "precious" ingredient of milk, it has been increasingly mixed with a wide variety of processed foods, including children's foods, fresh cheese, ready-made soups and diet foods.

An allergy is the body's response to fight a substance that it considers dangerous to its health and survival. Scientists have discovered that the beta casein (a protein in whey) can trigger an immune response that may, in turn, cross-react with an antigen to cause an allergic reaction. The dramatic increase in allergies in the developed world has coincided with the proliferation of food products that contain whey. Is it just possible that the current "allergy epidemic" in the western world may well be closely related to the "miracle food" whey?

Pasteurization

Once milk is pasteurized (heat-treated), its natural enzyme population is destroyed. Yet the enzymes are needed to make the milk nutrients available to the body cells. Newly born calves die within six months when fed with pasteurized cow's milk. One can only imagine the turmoil that must be going on in the tiny intestinal tract of a baby who is fed pasteurized milk or sterilized milk formula. Babies usually develop colic, become bloated and chubby, discharge mucus, catch colds, suffer from frequent ear-infections, are restless, and cry a lot. The best approach is to breastfeed as long as possible, avoid dairy-based formulas altogether, use alternatives such as coconut milk (next to ideal), almond milk or rice milk, and give freshly mashed fruits, vegetables and rice when the baby is ready to eat solids.

Homogenization

Homogenization of milk involves the use of extremely high pressure and filters to break up the fat globules in milk into minute particles. When homogenized milk was introduced in 1932, the occurrence of atherosclerotic damage (build-up of plaque in the inner walls of the arteries) began to increase. It appears that when fat globules are forcibly broken up by mechanical means, it allows an enzyme associated with milk fat, known *as xanthine oxidase*, to become free and penetrate the intestinal wall. Once xanthine oxidase gets through the intestinal wall and into the bloodstream, it is capable of creating scar damage to the heart and arteries which, in turn, may stimulate the body to release cholesterol into the blood in an attempt to lay a protective fatty material on the scarred areas. The appearance of cholesterol created widespread speculation that it was the cause of heart disease and not the result. The xanthine oxidase process is slow and destructive. Most 10-year old children who have consumed homogenized milk have some form of atherosclerosis. There is a very high correlation between countries that drink homogenized milk and the occurrence of atherosclerosis.

Milk Hormone (BST)

Bovine somatotrophin (BST) is a hormone which, when fed to cows, can increase their milk yield by 20-30%. In the U.S., BST was licensed by the Food and Drug Administration (FDA) in 1994.

This effectively gave farmers the legal permission to treat their herds with the controversial hormone. The license was accompanied with a new labeling policy, previously unheard of in the U.S.. Traditional dairy farmers are prohibited from labeling their milk as "hormone free," while those using the hormone are not required to say that they use BST. Because uncontrolled hormone intake is linked to a number of serious health problems, there has been great concern in the dairy industry that informed consumers would avoid milk that was labeled as coming from dairies that use BST. Their pressure ensured the above legislation.

Cows naturally produce a certain amount of milk according to the demand from their offspring. The hormone-induced artificial increase of milk yield causes a number of diseases in dairy herds that are met by administering large quantities of antibiotics. The drug's poisons migrate into the milk and its products, adding to the health risks related to BST.

Alternatives to Cow's Milk

In a culture that is so accustomed to drinking cow's milk and using it in combination with other foods such as breakfast cereals, it is convenient to have some healthy alternatives.

- **Coconut Milk:** This delicious milk is so rich in essential nutrients that it can be compared with human mother's milk. Many infants were raised with coconut milk when breast milk was not available. If fresh coconut milk cannot be obtained, you can use dried shredded coconut and blend it with water. Then press or strain through a cheese cloth or sieve. You may make enough coconut milk to last for up to 5 days. Keep refrigerated.
- **Almond milk:** This is one of the best and healthiest milk alternatives on the market today. It is available in most natural food stores and is starting to appear in an increasing number of grocery stores and supermarkets. Avoid buying brands that contain added vitamins and minerals. Almond milk will keep in

a refrigerator for about a week days after opening the container. For maximum shelf life, it is a good idea to refrigerate overnight before opening the sealed container. It is relatively easy to make almond milk in a good blender. Soak the almonds overnight to soften them, then blend and strain with cheesecloth. Using a commercial soymilk-maker is the fastest way of making almond milk.

- **Oat milk**: Although perhaps not as ideal as almond milk, oat milk is a reasonably good alternative to cow's milk. It is available in most places where almond milk is sold. It is a good idea to check the label before buying, as some of the oak milk brands currently on the market are actually a blend, containing milk from other grains and beans.
- **Rice milk**: Rice milk is also a reasonably good milk alternative. It is more apt to have additives to enhance the flavor, so it is a good idea to check the label.
- **Soy milk**: Like other soy products, soy milk should be avoided due to its natural food toxins, enzyme inhibitors, a possible gene-manipulation, and its potentially harmful effects on hormonal balance.

Chapter 13

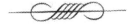

Sugar and Sweeteners

The consumption of sugar and artificial sweeteners has increased dramatically in recent years. If one were to plot the increase of sugar consumption year by year alongside the increase in obesity, immune disorders, blood-sugar disorders and a variety of other ailments, one would find similar growth curves. Sugar and sweeteners are undoubtedly not the only reason for declining health trends, especially among young people, but they are certainly a major contributor.

Sugar

Refined sugar is rapidly absorbed into the bloodstream. The resulting increase in blood sugar level causes the pancreas to secrete insulin in an effort to restore balance. It also stimulates the adrenal glands to secrete adrenalin in an effort to remove the sugar from the bloodstream. Adrenalin levels can increase by as much as 4 times, causing a stress response sometimes referred to as an "adrenalin rush." Afterwards, the blood sugar level drops below normal, which often leads to a state of depression, lethargy and irritability, sometimes referred to as the "sugar blues." In the long term, this can lead to various blood sugar disorders, such as diabetes and hypoglycemia.

This stress response also causes an increase in the production of both cholesterol and cortisone. Cortisone inhibits the immune functions, making a person much more vulnerable to colds, the flu, and other ailments. Neutrophils are one of five types of white blood cells that play a key role in the immune system. A study published in the December 1976 issue of *Dental Survey* investigated sugar's effect on neutrophils. This experiment found that consuming 24 ounces (2 cans) of cola depresses neutrophil activity by 50%. This occurs within 30 minutes after ingesting the cola and lasts for at least 5 hours, possibly longer. Other parts of the immune system may be similarly assaulted by sugar.

Refined sugar lacks vitamins and minerals and must draw upon the body's micro-nutrient stores in order to be metabolized. When these stores are depleted, metabolism of fatty acids and cholesterol is impeded, causing obesity due to higher fatty acid storage and higher cholesterol levels.

In the past 20 years, sugar consumption has increased from 26 pounds to 135 pounds per person per year. In the early 1900's, the average per capita consumption was only about 5 pounds per year, equivalent to about a 2-week supply at current consumption levels. Obviously, only a very small percentage of this is added to our foods and beverages at the dinner table in the form of white granular sugar with which we are all familiar. Most of it is insidiously added to processed foods and beverages by food processing companies. Sugar may be found on food package labels under a variety of names such as Glucose, Fructose, Sucrose, Galactose, Maltose and Lactose.

Sugars are added to processed foods to appeal to the palate, without regard to their ultimate effect on the body. For example, most breakfast cereals are laden with sugar. Cereals are primarily protein, which the body cannot metabolize well in the presence of sugar. Sugar is also acid-forming, which then draws on the alkaline reserves within the body to maintain an appropriate acid/alkaline balance.

Aspartame

As more and more people have become aware of the health hazards of sugar, there has been a tendency to look for sugar substitutes. The most widely used artificial sweetener today is aspartame, known under trade names such as NutraSweet, Equal, Spoonful, Equal-Measure, Benevia and NatraTaste. Since the patent on it has now expired, it will undoubtedly show up on the market under a variety of new trade names.

The approval in the U.S. of aspartame for use in beverages and dry foods is one of the most disgraceful chapters of political influence, payoffs and corruption in the history of the Food and Drug Administration (FDA). As a member of the National Soft Drink Association, the Coca-Cola Company opposed FDA approval of aspartame for beverages. Their objections, running to several pages published in the Congressional Record of May 7, 1985, said aspartame is uniquely and inherently unstable and breaks down in the can. It decomposes into formaldehyde, methyl alcohol, formic acid, diketopiperazine and other toxins. In a study on 7 monkeys, 5 had severe seizures and one died – a casualty rate of 86%. In spite of this testimony, after aspartame was approved by the FDA, the Coca-Cola Company introduced Diet Coke, which is laden with aspartame. The story has all too many familiar parallels with the tobacco companies that, in spite of their full knowledge of the severe health risks of smoking, continue to manufacture and promote the use of cigarettes.

The European Common Market has at least banned aspartame for use in all children's products.

Aspartame contains three primary ingredients:

- 50% Phenylalanine
- 40% Aspartic acid
- 10% Methanol (wood alcohol)

Let's start with **methanol**. When a beverage containing aspartame is ingested, the methanol (wood alcohol) is distributed widely throughout the body, including the brain, muscles, fat and nerve tissues. It then metabolizes to formaldehyde, which enters the cells and binds to the proteins and DNA. Cytogenetic effects (changes in and injuries to the DNA) have been shown to result from formaldehyde. The nature of the injury involves breaking and then cross-linking within genetic materials which alters the cells. The ability of aspartame to cause such cellular mutations has been shown in studies. Increases in malignant brain tumors are suggested to be associated with aspartame use.

Next, let's consider the effects of **aspartic acid**. It significantly raises the blood plasma level of aspartate and glutamate. Too much aspartate and glutamate in the brain kills certain neurons by allowing the influx of too much calcium into the cells. This influx triggers excessive amounts of free radicals, which kill the cells. The neural cell damage that can be caused by excessive aspartate and glutamate is why they are referred to as "excitotoxins." They "excite" or stimulate the neural cells to death.

Phenylalanine is the third component of aspartame. It is an amino acid normally found in the brain. People with the genetic disorder, phenylketonuria, cannot metabolize phenylalanine. This leads to dangerously high levels of phenylalanine in the brain (sometimes lethal). It has been shown that ingesting aspartame, especially along with carbohydrates, can lead to excessive levels of phenylalanine in the brain, even in people who do not have phenylketonuria. Excessive levels of phenylalanine in the brain can cause serotonin levels in the brain to decrease, leading to emotional disorders such as depression. Even a single use of aspartame raises the blood's phenylalanine levels. In his testimony before the U.S. Congress November 3, 1987, Dr. Louis J. Elsas explained that high blood phenylalanine can be concentrated in parts of the brain, and is especially dangerous for infants and fetuses.

Recent Study

The results of an extensive study on the effects of aspartame on laboratory rats, conducted jointly by two distinguished research institutions in Bologna, Italy, were reported in November 2005. The study involved feeding rats food that contained varying amounts of aspartame. There were six separate test groups, ranging from rather potent dosages of aspartame, to extremely mild dosages. The test groups involved a total of 1,500 rats; half male and half female. The experiment ended with the death of the last rat at 159 weeks. At the death of each rat, examinations were made of all organs and various tissue samples. The test animals showed extensive evidence of malignant cancer, including lymphomas, leukemias and tumors at multiple organ sites in both males and females.

According to other researchers and physicians studying the adverse effects of aspartame, the following chronic illnesses can be triggered or worsened by ingesting aspartame: brain tumors, multiple sclerosis, epilepsy, chronic fatigue syndrome, Parkinsons's disease, Alzheimer's, mental retardation, lymphoma, birth defects, fibromyalgia and diabetes.

Under a Freedom of Information order, the FDA admitted that over 75% of all the complaints that it receives from consumers related to food additives involve aspartame!

Saccharin

Saccharin, the Latin word for "sugar," is a chemical that was discovered in 1879, and was the first artificial sweetener. It is 300 times sweeter than sugar and does not metabolize in the body, so it has no calories. Saccharin, which is derived from coal tar, has a very controversial history.

In 1907 it was banned for use in the United States by the forerunner of the FDA because of health concerns. But through some political maneuvering, the ban was lifted a short time later. From time to time throughout the following years, studies were conducted, mostly on laboratory animals, regarding the safety of saccharin. As a point of interest, although saccharin was used mainly by people attempting to control their weight, studies going as far back at 1947 showed that animals that were fed saccharin (in comparison to control groups) displayed *increases* in appetite and weight gain.

In 1977, a Canadian study spotlighted saccharin as a carcinogen, and in March of that year the FDA issued a ban on the use of saccharin in the United States. However, a month later, due to industry pressure, the ban was deferred for 18 months. But during that time, companies were required to print a health warning on any products that contained saccharin. The 18 month deferral became an indefinite deferral, and in the year 2000, The National Institute of Health removed saccharin from its list of carcinogens, and Congress agreed to remove the warning requirement from products containing it.

Saccharin continues to be available as little pink packets of Sweet'N Low in most restaurants, and is still used as an artificial sweetener in an array of food products. For example, Diet Coke and Diet Pepsi use a blend of saccharin and aspartame, as does Tab.

Healthy Sweeteners

A bit of sweetness is not out of place in a healthy diet so long as it is in balance with other foods. There are several natural sweeteners that have few, if any, harmful side effects. However, just as sweet fruits and fruit juices need to be consumed in moderation, and in appropriate relationship to other types of foods, the same is true of the following natural sweeteners.

Honey

Honey is the oldest known natural sweetener, with references to it dating back virtually as far as recorded history. As we know, it is produced by bees from the nectar they collect from the blossoms of plants and trees. The color, flavor and scent of a particular honey is determined by the nectar of the flower from which it was collected, as well as the soil, its location, and the time of the year in which it was collected. In commercial bee-keeping operations, beehives are typically placed in close proximity to a natural source of nectar, such as a clover field or orange grove. The qualities of such honey are then predominately related to the clover or orange blossoms, but all honey is a blend of the nectar of various blossoms as bees follow their instincts in the gathering process.

The general rule of thumb is that the darker the honey, the more intense its flavor.

Honey has an enzyme system that produces hydrogen peroxide, a bactericidal agent that helps fight off infection. This is the same enzyme system that enables honey to keep without refrigeration.

Most honey is gently heated to enable filtering our of the wax and other agents. But the temperatures are kept low (less than 96° F) in order to preserve its enzymes and other nutrients. Such "raw" honey tends to crystallize over a period of time, so much of the honey found in grocery stores and supermarkets has been pasteurized to prevent crystallization. Unfortunately, this destroys the enzymes and many of its inherent nutrients. Therefore, it is much better to find a local source of raw honey.

Honey contains various disease-inhibiting antioxidants, similar to some common sweet fruits. Studies have shown that consumption of honey raises the level of antioxidants in the blood. There has been speculation that eating honey derived from plants in the local area in which one lives helps to fend off seasonal pollen-related allergies, but we are not aware of any studies that have explored this possibility.

Whereas most sweeteners are acid-forming when metabolized in the body, honey is moderately alkaline-forming.

Honey also has valuable properties as a healing agent when applied topically to wounds or various skin ailments. This is discussed in more detail in the book, *Timeless Secrets of Health and Rejuvenation*.

Xylitol

In spite of its ominous-sounding name, Xylitol is a natural carbohydrate that is found in fibrous plants and vegetables, including birch and other hardwood trees, berries, almond hulls and corncobs. It has been approved for use as a sugar substitute in over 35 countries. Xylitol is a sugar alternative that looks and tastes like real sugar, but contains less than 40% of the calories.

The human body produces small amounts (5-15 grams per day) during normal metabolism. In contrast to ordinary sugar, Xylitol does not encourage growth of yeast, including candida albicans. Xylitol also increases the absorption of B-vitamins and calcium.

Xylitol has been shown in studies to reduce dental decay up to 80% by neutralizing plaque acids and inhibiting the growth of Streptococcus mutant, the plaque-producing bacteria most responsible for causing dental cavities. Recent studies at the Dental Schools of Michigan and Indiana Universities have tested the effect of Xylitol/Sorbitol blends in chewing gum and mints on plaque. They showed a significant decrease in plaque accumulation. Xylitol also stimulates remineralization of tooth enamel.

Xylitol enjoys wide acceptance in Japan and the Scandinavian countries. In Russia it has been used for decades as a sweetener for diabetics, and in Germany in solutions for intravenous feeding. In the United States, Xylitol is approved as a direct food additive for special dietary uses. Numerous clinical and field studies performed over the past 30 years have demonstrated the safety and efficacy of Xylitol as a healthy alternative to sugar and artificial sweeteners. It can be purchased in bulk form from health food stores and many online sources.

Stevia

Stevia is an herb, native to Paraguay, that has been used as a sweetener and flavor enhancer for centuries. The Guarani Indians had known about the unique advantages of this plant long before the arrival of the Spanish invaders. Prior to 1900, stevia had grown only in the wild, and consumption was limited to those having access to its natural habitat. With the gradual introduction of stevia as a commercial crop, it eventually began to attract attention throughout Latin America and beyond.

Originally introduced to Japan in 1970, stevia-based products quickly caught on, and by 1981 reportedly represented 41% of the market share of potently sweet substances consumed in that country. Introduction in the United States has had a more difficult go of it because of strong lobbying resistance by the sugar industry. Since the passage of the Dietary Supplement Health and Education Act (DSHEA), stevia can be sold legally in the United States, but only as a "dietary supplement." The FDA will not permit it to be called a "sweetener" or even referred to as "sweet." In view of the aspartame debacle, this seems more than a bit ludicrous.

Numerous studies on the safety of stevia have been conducted in Japan and elsewhere, but no adverse side effects have ever been found.

Stevia is usually marketed in the U.S. as an extract, either in liquid or powder form. It can be found in most health and natural food stores – usually on the same shelf that contains other sweeteners, in spite of the FDA!

Stevia can also be grown as an herb in a wide range of climates. Although non-toxic, stevia plants have been found to have insect-repelling tendencies. One challenge for those attempting to grow stevia is that, like sesame, the seeds do not germinate as easily as most other plant seeds. Nevertheless, stevia plants are available from a variety of agricultural supply sources.

Caution: If you experience diarrhea after ingesting stevia, you may have be eating too much of it.

Other Natural Sweeteners

There are other sweeteners that deserve consideration. Most "natural" sweeteners are certainly preferable to refined sugar or chemical sweeteners.

Date sugar is a powder made by grinding up dried dates, so it enjoys the same health benefits as dates. However, date sugar does not dissolve well in liquids.

Pure maple syrup is made from the sap of sugar maple trees. Although it has a wonderful flavor, the boiling process used to thicken it damages many of its natural nutrients.

Agave syrup is made from the agave (uh-gah-vay) plant which has long been cultivated in hilly, semi-arid soils of Mexico. Its fleshy leaves cover the pineapple-shaped heart of the plant, which contains a delicious, sweet sticky juice, made of 90% fructose.

Chapter 14

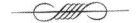

Unhealthy Beverages

There are many types of processed beverages widely available that are not particularly healthy for the body. This chapter will focus on three categories of beverages that have the most devastating effects on human health: soft drinks, alcoholic beverages and coffee.

Soft Drinks

The caffeine contained in most soft drinks (Mountain Dew, Coke, Pepsi, etc.) and most power drinks not only stimulates and stresses the central nervous system and immune system, but also acts as a powerful diuretic. For every can of cola you drink, you relinquish up to three times as much water – water that your body cannot afford to give up without suffering some sort of damage. Caffeine removes water from the body faster than the body can absorb it again, thereby generating constant thirst. People who frequently drink soft drinks are never able to really quench their thirst because their bodies continually run out of cellular water. There are some people who drink as many as 10-15 cans of cola a day. Eventually, they tend to confuse their body's never-ending thirst signal with hunger, and they begin to overeat, causing excessive weight gain.

Caffeine, being a nerve toxin, stimulates the adrenal glands to secrete stress hormones and trigger a strong immune response that may give the false impression that this newly found energy was derived from the consumed beverage. The secret behind these energizing stimulants is that the resulting immune reaction mobilizes enough energy for you to feel perked up and clear-headed, at least for as long as your body remains stimulated. To remove the nerve toxin, caffeine, from the blood, the body has to come up with extra water that the caffeine robs from its cells. This results in cellular dehydration and a temporary thinning of the blood.

Apart from its diuretic action and addictive effects on the brain, regular caffeine intake over-stimulates the heart muscles, causing exhaustion and risk of heart disease.

Unfortunately, caffeine is not the only culprit in soft drinks. Because of the sugars, artificial flavors and sweeteners contained in soft drinks, they are extremely acidic. It would take 32 glasses of alkaline water at an alkaline pH of 9 to neutralize the acid from just one 12 oz. cola or soda. In response to ingesting a cola, the body needs to use reserves of its own stored alkaline buffers – mainly calcium from the bones and DNA – in order to maintain proper blood alkaline pH levels. Acidic blood levels are a leading cause death! There are enough acids in one soda to kill you if your body didn't possess a mechanism to neutralize them. Over the long term, excessive consumption of soft drinks leads to a risk that the body will succumb to acidosis as mineral buffers become depleted.

There are approximately 8 to 9 teaspoons of sugar in a 12-oz. can of Coke, Pepsi or other well-known soft drinks. Because sugar is absorbed into the bloodstream so quickly, the blood sugar level rises dramatically. This causes the pancreas to secrete insulin in order to compensate for the excessive blood sugar. And it stimulates the adrenal glands to secrete adrenalin in an effort to remove sugar from the bloodstream. Adrenalin levels can increase by as much as four times normal, creating a state of "fight or flight" stress response within the body. Many people experience this as a boost of energy that they believe they are getting from the soft drink, but it is anything but that. This stress reaction also increases the production of both cholesterol and cortisone. Cortisone inhibits the immune functions, making one much more vulnerable to colds, the flu and other disorders. Afterwards, the blood sugar level drops below normal, which often leads to a state of depression, lethargy and irritability, sometimes referred to as the "sugar blues." In the long term, this can lead to various blood sugar disorders, such a diabetes or hypoglycemia.

Many people, aware of the adverse effects of sugar, opt for so-called "diet" drinks, such as Diet Coke or Diet Pepsi. Unfortunately, this can lead to even worse health complications. The sweetener that is most commonly used in diet soft drinks is aspartame. The health risks related to aspartame are discussed in Chapter 13.

In addition to the above risks, many soft drinks contain excessive amounts of the chemical Benzene, a poison that has been confirmed as a human carcinogen (cancer-causing agent) by the International Agency for Research on Cancer, the Department of Health and Human Services (DHHS), and the Environmental Protection Agency (EPA).

Alcoholic Beverages

When a person drinks an alcoholic beverage, about 20% of the alcohol is absorbed in the stomach, with the remaining 80% being absorbed in the small intestine. The alcohol then enters into the bloodstream and circulates throughout the body. As alcohol enters the nerve cells within the brain, it interferes with communication between the nerve cells and all other cells. The excitatory nerve pathways are suppressed, while the inhibitory pathways are stimulated. This has the effect of causing sluggishness of the body, which is characteristic of the behavior of someone who is under the influence of alcohol.

Depending on the level of alcohol within the bloodstream, certain centers of the brain are affected more than others. The first center to be affected is the cerebral cortex, which is why rational thinking tends to become blurred. As the alcohol level rises, it begins to affect the limbic system, involving our emotions and autonomic nervous system. The next center in the brain to be affected is the cerebellum, which among other things, affects our spatial orientation. This is why intoxicated people have difficulty walking in a straight line. And, if the alcohol level continues to increase, the next center to be impacted is the hypothalamus and pituitary gland, which together control the entire endocrine system of the body. And finally, excessive alcohol in the bloodstream reaches the medulla (brain stem), acting as a depressant on the entire central nervous system.

The body's natural defense mechanisms attempt to eliminate alcohol from the bloodstream in three different ways:

- The kidneys eliminate about 5% of the alcohol through the urine.
- The lungs eliminate about 5% through the breath, which can be detected through a breathalyzer device.
- The liver chemically breaks down the remaining alcohol into acetic acid.

As discussed in Part 1 of this book, the liver has a wide range of responsibilities related to keeping the body healthy. It functions according to a system of priorities, giving its attention to the most dangerous threats to the body first. Since alcohol is so toxic to the body, it assigns a high priority to the task of breaking it down so that it can be eliminated from the body. But while it is doing this task, other functions of the liver must take a back seat and wait their turn. So regular consumption of alcoholic beverages inhibits the ability of the liver to carry out its normal health-maintenance functions.

Excessive consumption of alcoholic beverages over a long period of time usually leads to alcoholic liver diseases, such as hepatitis and cirrhosis. Essentially these diseases involve a build-up of scar tissue within the liver, inhibiting its ability to function properly. In acute cases, the liver actually atrophies, often leading to death.

Alcohol, like caffeine, severely dehydrates the body. In fact, an alcoholic "hangover" is the result of dehydration of the cells of the brain. When alcohol enters the bloodstream, it causes the pituitary gland to block the creation of vasopressin. Without this chemical, the kidneys send water directly to the bladder, rather than reabsorbing it into the body. Studies have shown that consuming 250 milliliters of an alcoholic beverage causes the body to expel as much as 1,000 milliliters of water from the body.

And, also like caffeine, alcohol is extremely acidic. So it, too, draws on the alkaline reserves in the body in order to maintain an appropriate acid/alkaline balance.

In addition to the effects of alcohol, there are two alcoholic beverages that deserve special attention: beer and wine.

Beer

In addition to the issues related to the alcoholic content of beer, other factors are involved. A primary ingredient in the beer making process is hops. The hop plant is a member of the hemp family, and consequently a first cousin of cannabis, otherwise known as marihuana. The relaxing effect that beer has on those who consume it is derived from the hops ingredient hopein, which is a form of morphine. Hops also are known to function as an anti-aphrodisiac, suppressing sexual drive and performance in men.

Hops also contain the female sex hormones daidzein and genistein, which are commonly used to fatten calves, sheep and chickens. Beer also contains another female hormone, estrogen, which is found in a woman's ovaries. The typical "beer belly" and breast growth of a beer drinker is caused by these female hormones, and has little to do with beer calories.

The malt in beer also has a substance in it that influences the psyche; it is called hordenin. Hordenin results from the germination of barley, and is related to the well-known stimulants ephedrine and mescaline. It also has a strong diuretic effect, which compounds the dehydration of the body caused by the alcohol.

Wine

The wine industry tends to promote the idea that drinking a glass or two of red wine each day provides a benefit to your arteries. But this is misleading. A group of natural substances found in many kinds of foods, called flavonoids, seem to have powerful anti-clotting properties. They are amply present in purple grape juice and, to a lesser extent, in red wine. A 1999 study done at the University of Wisconsin Medical School found that red wine does, indeed, slow the activity of blood platelets by about 45%. But the study also showed that purple grape juice dampens them by about 75%. In other words, if you turn purple grape juice into wine, it loses some of the potency of its flavonoids. So to have the benefits advocated for red wine, it is far better to drink the fresh juice of purple grapes. There are about 4,000 different flavonoids found in natural plants. So eating a diet rich in fruits and vegetables is one of the best ways to maintain a healthy circulatory system; wine, with its substantial alcohol content, is not.

Coffee

The primary health risk associated with coffee is its high caffeine content – about 170 milligrams in a regular cup of coffee. Caffeine is a strong diuretic, and the manner in which caffeine tends to dehydrate the body has already been discussed. And, coffee is highly acid-forming, which means that it draws heavily on the alkaline reserve within the body in order to maintain a safe acid/alkaline balance.

Studies have shown that in North America, approximately 85% of adults drink 3 to 5 cups of coffee per day. Since it is a $90 billion industry, concerted efforts are made to downplay the health risks associated with coffee.

One of the incentives for drinking coffee is its perceived ability to serve as a stimulant when one's energy level starts to drop. But since coffee has no real energy of its own, just stimulants, where is the stimulated energy coming from? Obviously, the body is providing it. Stimulants are nerve toxins that trigger a powerful defense reaction in the body. This immune response is what one experiences as a boost in energy when one drinks a cup of coffee. So in reality, the energy boost that one experiences is actually an energy loss for the body. Repeated stimulation by drinking coffee through the day tends to deplete the energy reserve within the body.

If caffeine is the primary ingredient in coffee, and coffee is harmful to health, then what about decaffeinated coffee – does this eliminate the health risks? A recent study was conducted that involved three groups of people: one group drank regular coffee, another group drank decaffeinated coffee, and a third group drank no coffee. The results were reported at a November, 2005 meeting of the American Heart Association. The primary difference noted among the three groups was that those who drank decaffeinated coffee developed a higher level of blood fat associated with harmful LDL cholesterol. The reason is not entirely clear. The decaffeination process tends to destroy some of the flavonoids that give coffee its flavor. So decaffeinated coffee is usually made from a different type of coffee bean that has a more robust flavor. In light of this, the differences found in the study may relate to the different types of beans that were used, or to the decaffeination process itself.

It should also be noted that many people add sugar or artificial sweeteners to their coffee before drinking it. These additives carry their own health risks, as discussed in the previous chapter.

In the October, 2005 issue of *American Journal of Epidemiology*, Danish researchers reported the effects of coffee on pregnant women. The study found that women who drank 4 to 7 cups of coffee daily while pregnant had a 33% higher risk of fetal death. Further, they found that pregnant women who drank 8 or more cups of coffee a day had a 59% greater risk of fetal death. The association between coffee and fetal deaths was strongest after 20 weeks gestation.

It is interesting to note that there are numerous health conditions for which doctors routinely advise their patients to eliminate coffee and all caffeine from their diet. Among these are:

- Heart disease and heart palpitations
- High blood pressure
- High cholesterol

- Insomnia and interrupted sleep patterns
- Candida or yeast infections
- Chronic fatigue syndrome
- Migraines or other vascular headaches
- Osteoporosis
- Ulcers, heartburn and stomach problems
- Liver disease and gallbladder problems, such as gallstones
- Kidney or bladder problems, including kidney stones
- Diabetes or hypoglycemia

This evokes an obvious question: if it is important to eliminate coffee and caffeine from one's diet after one develops such health conditions, is it just possible that coffee and caffeine may have contributed to the development of the condition in the first place?

Chapter 15

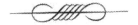

Vitamins and Minerals

The history of vitamins is related to a disease called beriberi, which was pervasive in Asia during the 19th century. By the year 1860, over one third of Japan's marines had fallen ill with symptoms such as weakness, weight loss and heart problems. The symptoms quickly disappeared whenever rice, Japan's most important staple food, was replaced with other foods.

Many years later, the Dutch physician Christiaan Eijkman, who was searching for the cause of beriberi, noted an interesting peculiarity. The chickens at the station where he was doing his work suddenly started to develop symptoms similar to beriberi. Upon further investigation, he found that these chickens were normally fed brown rice. But there had been a delay in the shipment of brown rice, so in the interim, the person responsible for feeding the chickens had been substituting white rice. When the next shipment arrived, and the chickens were returned to a diet of brown rice, the symptoms disappeared. Assuming that the white rice must be missing an important nutrient, Eijkman eventually discovered a few previously unknown substances within the bran of the brown rice; one of them he named B1.

This initiated the era of "vitamins," a term that includes the same root word as "vitality." This association of vitamins with vitality has become ingrained within our consciousness.

It eventually turned out that beriberi was not even caused by vitamin B1 deficiency. It should have been noticed from the beginning that people no longer suffered from beriberi once they discontinued eating rice altogether. In 1891, a Japanese researcher finally discovered that beriberi was caused by the poison citreoviridine. Citreoviridine is produced by mold in white rice that is stored in contaminated and humid environments. Yet even today, the vitamin B1 hypothesis as the cause of beriberi is still maintained in medical text books around the world.

Throughout the past century, scientists and nutritionists have added to the body of knowledge about vitamins. Thanks to their efforts, we now know that vitamins are organic compounds that are effective in minute amounts. Vitamins support essential processes in the body such as metabolism, growth and repair. Though we need only very small amounts of a wide variety of vitamins, a deficiency can produce symptoms associated with disease.

The best source of vitamins is natural foods, such as vegetables, fruits, nuts, seeds and grains. Such foods contain all of the vitamins that we need for optimal health, in appropriate combinations and forms that can easily be assimilated into our bodies. However, with the proliferation of processed foods, in which virtually all of the vitamins have been destroyed, researchers began to explore the possibility of creating synthetic vitamin "supplements" to be taken separately, and vitamin "additives" to be incorporated into processed foods. Although this has been an effective marketing ploy, to be able to promote foods as being "enriched" with vitamins, both vitamin supplements and additives have led to a wide range of health complications.

First and foremost, no one really knows how much of each vitamin we need. Governments and international organizations such as the World Health Organization frequently release figures that propose a Recommended Daily Allowance (RDA) for every vitamin that you supposedly need to stay healthy. The nutritional experts in different countries, however, have varying opinions about how much of each vitamin your body needs each day. An American, for example, is supposed to take at least 60mg of vitamin C, whereas a British citizen is considered better off taking only 30mg. People living in France need 80mg of this vitamin to stay healthy, whereas Italians are told they must consume approximately 45mg. These figures are "adjusted" every few years, even though our bodies' basic nutritional requirements have not changed.

To further confuse the issue, in recent years a new measurement scale has emerged known as Optimum Daily Allowance (ODA). Proponents of the new system argue that RDA is based on the *minimum* acceptable levels, rather than *optimal* levels. But the truth is, nobody really knows how much of each vitamin is good for us because the requirements, constitutions and absorption rates for vitamins differ from person to person.

Contrary to popular belief, individual vitamins do not have isolated functions. They work as a "team" within the body. Taking vitamins in supplemental form, rather than from natural foods, may be counter-productive since an excess of one vitamin can have a suppressing effect on another. Individual vitamins that have been isolated and extracted from foods can stimulate your nervous system. Feeling "energized," you naturally assume these vitamins must be good for you – that they must be increasing your "vitality." But stimulants never give you extra energy, they only force the body to spend and give up energy. Also, taking extra vitamins can be harmful if the body is unable to make use of them. Because vitamins are strong acids, an overload can lead to vitamin "poisoning," known as vitaminosis, which can be harmful to the kidneys.

Hidden Perils of Vitamin Pills

Following are a few examples of how taking various vitamin supplements can be detrimental to your health.

Vitamin A

It is a well known fact that too much vitamin A can cause deformities in unborn children. For this reason, there is a law prohibiting the addition of this vitamin to foods. Yet this law does not apply to animal feeds, even though it is well established that vitamin A accumulates in the liver of farm animals. Pregnant women are usually warned *not* to consume liver in order to avoid potential damage to their babies. If consuming extra vitamin A is considered dangerous for pregnant women or unborn babies, it cannot be considered safe for the rest of the population either.

Vitamin B

This is not a single vitamin, but rather an array of substances that have been categorized within the vitamin B series. Following are some of the health issues related to three of the substances within this group:

- **Vitamin B3**

  More commonly knows as **niacin**, vitamin B3 is one of the most popular B-vitamins. Now added to a large number of processed foods, including breakfast cereals, niacin is not without risks. After large doses of niacin (3g) had been given to patients suffering from psychiatric diseases, many developed hepatitis and other liver problems. Among other symptoms of niacin poisoning are hot flushes, itching skin, arrhythmia and nervousness. Illegal use of niacin in meats such as hamburger has often led to similar symptoms. The main reason for adding niacin to meat is to color it red and give it the appearance of being fresh. If you experience symptoms such as hot flashes after eating meat, then you are likely to have been poisoned with niacin.

- **Vitamin B6**

  Also known as **pyridoxin**, vitamin B6 is a combination of six substances. It has often been used as a drug to treat depression, pre-menstrual tension, schizophrenia and child asthma. It was considered safe until 1983 when scientists discovered a syndrome related to circulatory problems in the hands and feet of a number of patients who were given large doses of vitamin B6. The patients developed symptoms similar to the ones caused by the drug thalidomide. Some mothers who had taken large amounts of B6 during their pregnancy also reported deformities in their children's bodies. It took a long time before the nerve damage was linked to vitamin B6 poisoning. As it turned out, many patients who had been diagnosed with Multiple Sclerosis also had been poisoned by vitamin B6. There are many unsuspecting people currently taking vitamin B6 without any awareness of the risks involved.

- **Vitamin B9**

This vitamin is perhaps better known as **folic acid**. It is a common food additive, and potentially one of the most harmful ones. After researchers first discovered that people in malaria regions tended to have a deficiency of folic acid, they gave them this B vitamin in the belief that it would make their immune systems more resistant to the malaria virus. The children who were given this vitamin felt worse after the treatment, and were found to have much higher concentrations of malaria-causing agents in their blood than before taking the vitamin. The explanation for this phenomenon is that the malaria virus requires large amounts of folic acid in order to spread. People who have a deficiency in this vitamin are being naturally protected from malaria infection.

After discovering that children who took folic acid developed malaria, a British doctor in Kenya gave folic acid to one group of monkeys and compared them with another group of monkeys who were folic acid deficient. All the monkeys given folic acid supplements became infected with malaria, whereas the ones with "abnormally low" levels stayed healthy.

Over 40 percent of the world's population is threatened by malaria today, which is no longer restricted to developing countries. Malaria is rapidly becoming the leading cause of death in the world. One can only imagine the disastrous consequences that may have arisen from giving millions of healthy people vitamins to help their assumed vitamin deficiency. What is considered to be a vitamin deficiency for one person may be a life-saving response for another person.

Vitamin C

The most popular of all vitamins is **ascorbic acid,** or vitamin C. A deficiency of vitamin C is believed to cause hemorrhages, anemia, scurvy (damage of blood vessels), and to slow wound healing. It is, in fact, very easy to cure scurvy with red peppers, citrus fruits or cranberries, all of which contain high concentrations of vitamin C. Since the Hungarian scientist Szent Gyoerkyi identified vitamin C in oranges to be an effective substance for curing scurvy, it became a common assumption that vitamin C and orange juice must have the same benefits. But as it turned out, scurvy cannot be cured by vitamin C alone. Regardless of how large a dosage of vitamin C you use, the blood vessels will remain damaged. By contrast, eating a few oranges or red peppers cures scurvy quickly, without a trace of damage remaining. Fruits that are rich in vitamin C contain another ingredient that is known as vitamin C2. Scurvy can only be cured if vitamin C and vitamin C2 are taken together. When Gyoerkyi studied vitamin C, he included both compounds (C+C2). But as the years passed, the scientific community began omitting C2, and today there is very little awareness of it.

When vitamins became popular in the United States, there was a sudden jump in the number of newly born babies developing scurvy. It had previously been thought that scurvy had been eradicated a long time ago. As this mysterious development was investigated, it was discovered that the mothers of the affected babies had taken extra vitamin C preparations (without C2) in the belief that it was good for their babies. Faced with the supplemental dosages of vitamin C, the mothers' bodies started eliminating more of it than they ingested. When the babies were born they also continued removing whatever vitamin C they had received from the mother, because this is what they had learned to do while in the womb. Since their baby food did not contain significant amounts of vitamin C, they soon developed the dangerous baby scurvy.

The body of an adult who consumes vitamin C regularly may eventually produce a similar response. They may even develop scurvy because the body becomes programmed to eliminate vitamin C faster and in larger quantities than it is ingested. It is not uncommon for adults who have been taking vitamin C regularly to develop further complications if they suddenly stop taking it.

The November 2004 issue of the *American Journal of Clinical Nutrition* reported that according to new research, older women with diabetes who take high doses of vitamin C for the sake of their hearts may be doing more harm than good. The study, which followed nearly 2,000 postmenopausal women with diabetes for 15 years, found that those who took heavy doses of vitamin C supplements – 300 milligrams a day or more – were approximately twice as likely to die of heart disease or stroke compared with women who took no supplemental vitamin C. Interestingly, those with a high intake of vitamin C from natural foods did not increase their risk of death from cardiovascular causes.

Vitamin D

Calciferol, known as vitamin D, is not a vitamin in the sense that, unlike other vitamins, the body is capable of producing it. With the help of UV light from the sun, the body synthesizes it from cholesterol in the human skin. Vitamin D, which acts more like a hormone than a vitamin, facilitates the absorption and utilization of calcium and phosphorus, necessary for maintaining strong bones and teeth. Although vitamin D levels cannot be influenced through diet, the nutritional textbooks indicate 2.5 micrograms as the daily requirement of this vitamin for adults.

Breast milk is considered to have deficiencies in vitamin D, implying that nature made a crucial mistake when it invented breast milk. Mothers are warned that, without taking extra amounts of this important vitamin, their babies could risk contracting rickets or developing bone deformities. Yet mothers are rarely informed about the risks involved when they overuse vitamin D. Vitamin D poisoning leads to something very similar to rickets.

Dr. Ernst Lindner, of the University of Giessen in Germany, has warned that if large amounts of vitamin D are given to a person, calcium is removed from the bones. He also states that it is very risky to add vitamin D to food. Bone deformation is more likely to occur in babies who are *not* breast-fed. Until the vitamin D pill came on the market, rickets in babies was effectively treated with breast milk. Nature deemed it necessary to supply mother's milk with only very small amounts of vitamin D. Studies have shown that the vitamin D content in mother's milk does not increase when the mother takes vitamin D supplements. This implies that a mother's body filters out vitamin D to protect the baby from being poisoned by overdoses of this vitamin. A baby's body easily synthesizes vitamin D from sunlight once it is exposed to it. It is, therefore, unnecessary to have this vitamin present in the mother's milk. The major cause of vitamin D deficiency among babies is keeping them in dark rooms with little or no natural light. But even with less than adequate sun exposure, they are still capable of absorbing sufficient amounts of calcium from the blood that are necessary for the building of healthy bones.

What Constitutes a Vitamin Deficiency?

The vitamin euphoria has emerged in spite of the fact that there are no reliable methods to determine if or when someone is suffering from a vitamin deficiency. In view of the harmful effects caused by supplemental vitamin intake, it is likely that a deficiency, if it really exists, is either caused by an overtaxed digestive system or by overdosing the body with vitamins. Blood vessel wall congestion and intestinal problems inhibit vitamins from reaching the cells, tissues, organs and systems in the body. It is erroneous to assume that by taking extra vitamins the body will automatically make use of them. We simply do not know how much of the vitamin intake will leave the stomach unharmed, in what amounts the vitamins are going to be digested, and to what extent they are likely to be absorbed by the blood and the body's cells. There are no two people on the planet with exactly the same vitamin requirements and absorption rates. What may be normal for one person may not be normal for another, which makes the "standardized vitamin requirements for all" questionable, if not potentially harmful.

Minerals

Mineral salts that are found in the earth's soil and rocks are classified as inorganic, and must be incorporated within the structure of plants in order to be usable by the body. Most mineral supplements are inorganic, and their consumption can cause serious problems, as they commonly end up deposited in various tissues throughout the body. This can result in serious health problems including arthritis, Alzheimer's disease and arteriosclerosis. Calcium supplements are notorious for this. The best source of usable organic minerals is fresh raw vegetables, with fruit ranking second best. Some nuts and seeds are also abundant with minerals; for example, sesame seeds supply an enormous 1,160 milligrams of calcium per 100 grams of seeds.

Unlike vitamins, minerals cannot be synthesized by plants. Plants draw up mineral salts (inorganic compounds) from the soil and convert them into colloidal minerals (organic compounds). Even a healthy digestive system has difficulty absorbing inorganic minerals, and this problem is compounded if the small intestine is impacted with toxic waste material. In the case of a very healthy adult, the absorption rate for inorganic minerals is 3-5%; the rest merely passes through the body without benefit, but often not without causing harm. Although these minerals now come in chelated form, (amino acids or protein are wrapped around them to improve assimilation), they are still inorganic and of very little use to the cells of the body.

Ionic minerals, on the other hand, have an absorption rate of 98%, which indicates that only minerals in their organic (angstrom size) form are meant to be used by the human physiology (to obtain a good source of ionic minerals, see "Sources" at the end of the book). If the soil is not replenished with minerals after harvesting, it becomes increasingly mineral deficient. Modern methods of agriculture generally do not include putting minerals back into the soil. Before the era of continuous soil depletion, the topsoil contained as many as 90-100 different minerals. Plants with deep root systems, such as alfalfa, tend to be the best source of minerals.

The great rivers, such as the Nile in Egypt and the Ganges in India, caused extensive flooding every year, bringing new minerals from the glaciers and mountains to the land, automatically enriching it. The people living in these areas were generally in excellent health, sometimes living to an age of 120-140 years. The situation changed with the attrition of forests and building of dams. Today, there are merely 12-20 minerals found in plant foods. Modern chemical fertilizers (nitrogen, phosphorus and potassium) may be sufficient to raise normal looking crops; yet the healthy looking plants are deficient in minerals. This can lead to mineral deficiencies in the body. We are consistently missing out on the majority of minerals. And if the digestive system does not function efficiently, a health crisis may arise. Almost every disease today is linked to a deficiency of one or more minerals or trace minerals.

Taking supplements consisting of inorganic minerals is not only inefficient, because of their relatively low absorption rate, but also potentially toxic to the body.[3] To illustrate, let's examine in detail the body's reaction to self-treatment with high doses of synthetic iron pills. Adrenal glands are stimulated by the introduction of excess inorganic iron. As a reaction, sodium levels rise. Elevated sodium causes magnesium levels to plunge. This signals calcium levels to sink, which in turn causes the potassium level to jump. This, in turn, causes decreased levels of copper and zinc. The net result is a chemical imbalance capable of producing a host of symptoms from headaches to heart palpitations. Most significant, however, this chemical balancing act depletes iron further, leaving the body more anemic than before taking the iron supplements.

If, on the other hand, the anemic person had eaten an abundance of fresh, iron-rich foods such as leafy green vegetables, prunes, black raspberries and Bing cherries, the body would have absorbed all the organic iron it needed and excreted the excess. The body knows when to say "no" to iron in its natural, organic form; it can't always tell when to stop with a continuing barrage of synthetic supplements.

Summary

The best sources of vitamins and minerals are vegetables, fresh fruit, grains, legumes, nuts and seeds – the foods that nature provides us. By including a wide variety of these in our regular diet, we can be reasonably assured that our body will receive all of the vitamins and minerals that are needed. Most serious vitamin and mineral deficiencies are the result of consuming too many acid-forming processed foods and beverages. Attempting to compensate for the lack of healthy vitamins and minerals in such "dead" foods by depending on additives, or by taking supplements, is potentially dangerous, and can often lead to health problems that are more serious than the original deficiency.

Chapter 16

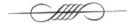

Foods with Special Health-Enhancing Qualities

Every plant has its own unique effect on the human body. While a few are poisonous, most impact the body in a much more positive way. The science of herbology deals with special healing effects of literally hundreds of different types of herbs.

Many of the fresh natural foods we find in the produce section of most modern grocery stores or supermarkets have special health-enhancing qualities in addition to their normal nutritional value.[9] A few of the more common ones will be discussed in this chapter. More extensive information can be found in *Timeless Secrets of Health and Rejuvenation*.[15]

Cautionary Note

Each of us is a unique human being. A particular food that is health-enhancing for one person may be unhealthy for another. And even for the same person, a food that may be beneficial to health today may have the opposite effect six months from now due to our continually changing body chemistry. If you are considering eating one of the following foods for the indicated benefits, it is advisable to first muscle test the food as described in Appendix A, to see if it would be appropriate for you at this time. Also, listen to the messages of comfort and discomfort that your body sends you in response to eating your food.

Broccoli's Anti-Cancer Properties

Small quantities of fresh broccoli sprouts contain as much cancer protection as larger amounts of the mature vegetable sold in food markets, according to researchers at Johns Hopkins University. For example, you would have to eat about two pounds of broccoli a week in order to reduce your risk of colon cancer by about 50%, whereas just 1 ounce of broccoli sprouts contains the same amount of cancer-inhibiting enzymes. Broccoli is also a super source of chromium that helps regulate insulin and blood sugar.

Cabbage – The Romans' Cancer Cure

Cabbage was revered in ancient Rome as a cancer cure. Today, we know its cancer-curing effects from its numerous anti-cancer and antioxidant compounds. Cabbage speeds up estrogen metabolism, which is thought to help block breast cancer and suppress the growth of polyps, a prelude to colon cancer. According to one study, eating cabbage more than once a week cut men's colon cancer odds by as much as 66%. Cabbage also contains powerful anti-ulcer compounds; its juice has been shown to help heal ulcers in humans. Red cabbage has twice the fiber as white cabbage and is known for its balancing effects on blood cholesterol.

Cauliflower Helps Fight Breast Cancer

Cauliflower contains many of the same cancer-fighting, hormone-regulating compounds as its cousins, broccoli and cabbage. Cauliflower is one of the least popular vegetables, but this does not make it less important. Researchers have found that it helps women break down estrogen and create estrogen by-products is a safe way, slashing breast cancer risk by 40%. It also helps ward off colon cancers.

The Great Carrot Phenomenon

Carrots are a rich source of beta carotene, a powerful anti-cancer, artery-protecting, immune-boosting and infection-fighting antioxidant. Recent research has shown that a single carrot a day slashed stroke rates in women by 68%! If you are or were a smoker, the beta-carotene in one medium-size carrot can cut your lung cancer risk in half. Your eyes will be grateful for that "carrot a day" as well. It has been shown that high doses of beta carotene, as found in carrots, substantially reduce the odds of degenerative eye diseases (cataracts and macular degeneration). It also helps moderate chest pain (angina). The high soluble fiber in carrots balances blood cholesterol and promotes regularity. Cooking carrots makes it easier for the body to absorb the beta-carotene.

Celery – Better Than Viagra

Celery has long been known as one of the best foods to keep your blood pressure normal. It dilates blood vessels like most potent drugs, but without the harmful side effects. Who would have thought, though, that this common food could turn out to be far more effective than Viagra or other sex-enhancing drug?

According to an exhaustive study of purported aphrodisiac foods, celery is the "sexiest" substance on earth. This unlikely-sounding candidate combines ideal amounts of vitamin E, magnesium, niacin, potassium and zinc – all required for optimum sex. And it gets even better. Celery contains arginine, a natural amino acid that expands blood vessels much like Viagra. Yet, unlike Viagra, arginine also increases blood flow to the clitoris and makes female genitals more responsive.

Celery is also an excellent source of vitamin C, a vitamin that helps to support the immune system. And it contains an ingredient, acetylenics, which has been shown to stop the growth of cancer cells. Celery is an excellent source of organic sodium, which gives it a slightly salty taste. Along with potassium, sodium helps to maintain the body's electrolyte balance. Just 4 stalks a day (or some celery juice) will do the trick.

Avocado – The Delicious Super Fruit

Avocado is a very dense fruit, packed with nutrients. It is especially rich in vitamin A, various B vitamins, calcium, iron, 9 essential amino acids, and high quantities of potassium. The avocado has been shown to benefit circulation, lower cholesterol and dilate blood vessels. It is true that avocados are high in fat – one reason they have earned the nickname "butter pear." But its primary fat, monounsaturated oleic acid (also concentrated in olive oil), acts as an antioxidant to block LDL cholesterol.

A 1996 study by researchers at the Instituto Mexicano del Seguro Social in Mexico looked at the health benefits of daily avocado consumption. The 45 subjects who ate avocados every day for just one week experienced an average of 17% drop in total blood cholesterol. Their cholesterol ratio also changed in a healthy way: their LDL (low-density lipoprotein) and triglycerides dropped significantly while their HDL (high-density lipoprotein) levels climbed.

Avocados have also been found to have three times the amount of glutathione than any other fruit. Glutathione is a powerful antioxidant shown to block 30 different carcinogens as well as the proliferation of the AIDS virus in test tube experiments. Studies have revealed a strong correlation between increased glutathione intake (from food) and decreased risk of oral and pharyngeal cancer.

Blueberries and Cranberries Protect
Kidneys, Heart, Eyes, Skin

Urinary tract infections (UTIs) are triggered by bacteria, primarily E. coli, adhering to the walls of the bladder or kidney. Many scientific studies have found that blueberries and cranberries are beneficial in fighting UTIs by blocking or prohibiting the growth of bacteria. Cranberry juice has traditionally been known to clear up a bladder infection or urinary tract infection within 1-2 days. It is recommended to take some juice 4 times per day, about one-half hour before meals and just before going to sleep.

Cranberries are an acid-forming food. So except for their therapeutic use, they should be eaten very sparingly. Because of their tart taste, sweeteners are usually added to make them more palatable. Since sugar is also highly acid-forming in the body, it definitely should not be added to cranberries as a sweetener.

Research shows that blueberries contain high concentrations of antioxidant compounds with beneficial medicinal properties. Blueberries' reported medicinal benefits include preventing urinary tract infections, stimulating anti-cancer activity, reducing heart disease risk, strengthening collagen, regulating blood sugar, improving night vision, reducing replication of the HIV virus, and treating diarrhea. Cranberries are rich in bioflavonoids and natural vitamin C that stimulate the immune system and fight off infection. Just eating more cranberries in the winter can ward off colds and flu.

In addition, cranberries can reduce the occurrence of kidney stones. They can also help dilate the bronchial tubes during an asthma attack. Cranberries are even beneficial for those suffering from acne, since they prevent acne-causing bacteria from entering the skin. So breakouts are less frequent and less severe.

The malic acid contained in cranberries helps soften stones in the bile ducts of the liver, and thus may be helpful in the preparatory phase of the liver cleanse. It is best to use a pure form of organic concentrate that can be diluted at the ratio of 1 part juice to 4 parts water.

The Healing Power in Green Beans

Also known as snap beans, green beans are loaded with nutrients of significant medicinal value. They are an excellent source of vitamin K, which is essential for maintaining strong bones. And they contain an abundance of other vitamins and minerals including: vitamin A, vitamin C, vitamin B_6, riboflavin, potassium, iron, manganese, folate, magnesium, thiamin, phosphorous, calcium, niacin, copper and zinc.

For atherosclerosis, diabetic heart disease and stroke, few foods compare to green beans in their number of helpful nutrients. Magnesium and potassium work together to help lower high blood pressure, while folate and vitamin B_6 help convert the potentially dangerous protein molecule homocysteine into other benign molecules. Homocysteine can directly damage blood vessel walls if not promptly converted; high levels are associated with a significantly increased risk of heart attack and stroke.

The iron content in green beans is twice as high as in spinach. This useful plant iron comes in ionic, organic form, unlike the toxic rust (iron oxide) contained in food supplements and breakfast cereals. Iron is an integral component of hemoglobin, which transports oxygen from the lungs to all body cells, and is also part of key enzyme systems for energy production and metabolism. To properly utilize iron for hemoglobin synthesis, the body requires copper, which is also amply present in green beans. Vitamins C and A, along with zinc, which are present in green beans help to maintain optimal immune function and acne-free skin. Last but not least, green beans help maintain your memory with thiamin (vitamin B_1).

Note: Green beans contain a measurable amount of oxalates. So if you suffer from oxalic acid stones in the kidneys, make certain to cleanse your kidneys before eating green beans on a regular basis.

The Bone Bone-Building Power of Brussels Sprouts

By age 70, one of every two women in the U.S. will likely suffer a painful fracture due to weak bones. Hip fractures are sometimes fatal. But, a recent woman's study shows that by eating Brussels sprouts, women can slash the risk of a hip fracture by 30%.

In addition, phytochemicals found in Brussels sprouts enhance the activity of the body's natural defense systems to protect against disease, including cancer. Scientists have found that sulforaphane, a potent phytonutrient contained in Brussels sprouts, boosts the body's detoxification enzymes. Brussels sprouts are also a good source of fiber and folate, and an excellent source of vitamin C. Vitamin C supports immune function and the manufacture of collagen, a protein that forms the basic substance of body structures including the skin, connective tissue, cartilage and tendons.

Artichoke for Good Digestion

The artichoke (Cynara scolymus) has been known for centuries for its beneficial effects on digestion. Its most noteworthy effect is increased bile production. Because the body uses cholesterol to make bile acids, increasing bile acid production may balance blood cholesterol. Increasing bile acid secretions also aids digestion – the reason why artichokes have traditionally been used for indigestion. Additionally, its leaves contain phytonutrients, that have numerous health-enhancing effects.

Kale

This nutritious vegetable comes in quite a few variations and colors – green and purple being the most common. It has been part of a traditional diet in parts of Africa where people live very long and healthy lives. Kale is a rich source of various anti-cancer chemicals. Being a member of the cruciferous family, it is endowed with anti-cancer indoles that help regulate estrogen and fight off colon cancer. It contains more beta carotene than spinach and twice as much lutein, the most of any vegetable tested. Kale is also high in antioxidants. Collard greens and other green leafy vegetables share similar benefits.

Nuts

In general, nuts have anti-cancer and heart-protective properties. Almonds and walnuts particularly help balance cholesterol levels. Both contain high concentrations of antioxidant oleic acid and mono-unsaturated fat, similar to that in olive oil, known to protect arteries from damage. Almonds, however, seem to be the more valuable of the two.

A total of six studies showed the resounding results of almonds' ability to lower total and LDL cholesterol, and reduce the risk of heart disease by 10%. All it takes is eating one small handful of almonds (1 ounce) a day. A good way to eat almonds is to soak them overnight so they can be digested more easily.

Nuts are generally high in antioxidant vitamin E, shown to protect against chest pain and artery damage. Brazil nuts are extremely rich in selenium, an antioxidant also linked to lower rates of heart disease and cancer. Walnuts contain ellagic acid, an antioxidant and cancer-fighter. Nuts are also good regulators of insulin and blood sugar, preventing steep rises. This makes them appropriate foods for those with glucose intolerance and diabetes. It is interesting to note that nuts have been found to be lacking in the diets of those who later develop Parkinson's disease.

Beware of allergies and rancid nuts. Nuts, particularly peanuts, are a prime cause of acute allergic reactions in susceptible individuals. Avoid nuts that are broken, chopped or in pieces, for they become rancid easily. Nut butters are also notorious for causing adverse reactions in the digestive system. When ground and thereby exposed to oxygen, they oxidize, i.e., become rancid. Rancid fats are very toxic and a major cause of illness. They may even lead to Crohn's disease.

Eat only fresh nuts. Avoid eating nuts that come mixed up with dried fruits (trail mix) or in commercially produced breakfast cereals; the nuts tend to be rancid and the dried fruits contain fungi.

Fresh Corn Can Help Reverse Vision Problems

Almost every person with age-related macular degeneration, which is the leading cause of blindness, suffers from lutein-deficiency. A recent study showed that consuming 6 mgs of lutein in your food per day reduces your risk of this disorder by a whopping 43%. Fresh corn is an excellent source of lutein.

Rice

This common food has anti-diarrheal and anti-cancer properties. Like other grains, rice contains anti-cancer protease inhibitors. Of all grains and cereals, it is the least likely to provoke bowel distress, such as intestinal gas or spastic colon. Whole rice is excellent for constipation, it lowers cholesterol and tends to block development of kidney stones. Basmati rice appears to have the highest nutritious value. It is a rich source of iron, selenium, thiamine and niacin. It also contains an ample amount of protein.

Coconut Oil – A Gift from the Tropics

Virgin coconut oil is rich in lauric acid, a proven antiviral and antibacterial agent. It is currently being used in treating AIDS. Lauric acid is also found in human mother's milk, which makes cococut milk an excellent alternative to milk-formula foods.

Delicious tasting coconut oil is not only satisfying to your taste buds, but it also cleanses your colon by gently softening and loosening old fecal material, and helping to remove it without unpleasant side effects. It has a strongly alkalizing effect in the body, which is beneficial for every disease process. This tropical oil contains a substance that has been shown to raise HDL cholesterol levels, the good kind, thereby lowering the risk of heart attack.

For those who are concerned about infestation with intestinal parasites and Candida albicans, coconut's anti-parasitic properties help purge pathogenic organisms by robbing them of their protective coating. A natural anti-yeast treatment, coconut oil has been known for many centuries to prevent yeast infections in women in the Pacific islands. During scientific tests, very large amounts of both capric and lauric acid, found in coconut oil, proved to be absolutely lethal to all major strains of Candida albicans.

Coconut oil also assists with dissolving and removing toxins that are trapped in fatty deposits, thereby making fat accumulation increasingly unnecessary. (Accumulation of fat is a survival mechanism to keep toxins engulfed within fatty tissue.) This may explain why coconut oil helps to build lean muscles. Many body builders, personal trainers, Olympic athletes and others use it for building lean body mass.

Coconut oil is easily digested, even by weak and compromised digestive systems. It assists with most digestive disorders, such as Crohn's disease and irritable bowel syndrome. This oil does not require any enzymes or carriers to be transported across cell membranes. Coconut oil is useful for the very young and the very old, alike. It is one of the healthiest and safest oils. Unlike most oils, however, coconut oil will not oxidize upon heating. This makes coconut oil the ideal cooking oil.

A Banana a Day Keeps the Doctor Away

When you compare it to an apple, the banana has four times the protein, twice the carbohydrates, three times the phosphorus, five times the vitamin A and iron, and twice the other vitamins and minerals. It is also rich in potassium and is one of the best value foods around. Bananas contain three natural sugars – sucrose, fructose and glucose – combined with fiber. In this form a banana gives an instant, sustained and substantial boost of energy. Research has shown that just two bananas can provide enough energy for a strenuous 90-minute workout.

Chapter 17

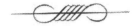

Microwave Cooking

Microwave cooking technology was originally developed in Nazi Germany in the early 1940's. The motivation for the development related to logistics of the war effort. If food for troops being deployed to distant locations could be cooked easily and quickly with microwave energy, it would eliminate the need to transport fuels needed for conventional ovens.

At the conclusion of the war, both the Russians and the Americans obtained microwave cooking equipment along with data from tests that had been conducted by the Germans. In Russia, extensive testing related to microwave cooking began about 1957. As the tests ensued, the mounting volumes of data related to the negative impact on human health were so disturbing that in 1974 Russia banned the use of microwaves for cooking in that country, and issued an international warning about its dangers.

The April 1992 *Journal of Pediatrics* reported that researchers at the Stanford University Medical Center discovered significant changes in human breast milk that was microwaved just enough to warm it. The changes included the destruction of 98% of its immunogloban-A antibodies and 96% of its liposome activity, which inhibits bacterial infections.

Dr. Lita Lee, of Hawaii, reported in the December 9, 1989 issue of *Lancet*: "Microwaving baby formulas converted certain trans-amino acids into their synthetic cis-isomers. Synthetic isomers, whether cis-amino acids or trans-fatty acids, are not biologically active. Further, one of the amino acids, L-proline, was converted to its d-isomer, which is known to be neurotoxic (poisonous to the nervous system) and nephrotoxic (poisonous to the kidneys). It's bad enough that many babies are not nursed, but now they are given fake milk (baby formula) made even more toxic via microwaving."

In 1991 there was a lawsuit in Oklahoma concerning a woman who had undergone a routine hip surgery. After the surgery, a blood transfusion was administered to her. Blood for transfusions is routinely warmed, but not in microwave ovens. In this particular case however, the nurse, unaware of the risks, *did* warm the blood in a microwave oven. The patient died 90 minutes after the transfusion. It seems obvious from this case that microwave ovens are doing something to substances other than warming them.

The concerns related to microwave cooking fall into 4 categories:

- The effects of microwave radiation on people who are in the vicinity of the microwave oven while it is being used.
- The potential negative impact on the nutritional value of food that has been cooked in a microwave oven.
- The potential of carcinogens and other health-endangering agents being created within the food as a result of being bombarded by microwave energy.
- The effects on human health as a result of eating food that has been cooked in a microwave oven.

Microwave Radiation

The dangers of microwave radiation are well known. The hazards first became apparent in conjunction with the development and use of radar, which utilizes bursts of microwave radiation at very high power levels. Until the effects were better understood, and appropriate precautions taken for workers in the vicinity of radar systems, microwave radiation resulted in numerous cases of severe illness and even death.

Although radiation standards have been established for the manufacture of microwave ovens, nobody really knows for certain what levels of radiation can be considered "safe." One thing that *is* known about the harmful effects of microwave radiation is that they are cumulative. So radiation levels that may be relatively "safe" based on infrequent or occasional use, may not be at all safe for someone who uses a microwave oven on a daily basis.

There are special dangers for pregnant women. A U.S. government agency has acknowledged that the human fetus is "probably the most sensitive segment of the population potentially exposed to radiation." Children represent another sensitive segment of the population.

The intensity of microwave radiation varies exponentially according to the distance from the source. The standard established in the U.S. in 1971 for maximum radiation "leakage" from a microwave oven is 1 milliwatt per square centimeter at a distance of 2 inches from the oven surface for new microwave ovens (prior to sale), and 5 milliwatts per square centimeter thereafter. At the 5 milliwatt level, the radiation would be down to 0.05 milliwatts at a distance of 20 inches, and only 0.005 millawatts at a distance of 5 feet. The message here is simple: NEVER stand close to a microwave oven when it is in operation. This is especially important for children.

Unfortunately, microwave ovens tend to be located in kitchens based on convenience, rather than safety. Oftentimes this means they are located at eye level, resulting in the greatest radiation exposure to the head. This is particularly disconcerting in view of the fact that one of the common effects of excessive microwave radiation reported by the Russians is a degeneration of brain circuitry and increased levels of disturbance in alpha-, delta-, and theta-wave signal patterns. Obviously, the safest alternative is to not even have a microwave oven in your house!

The Hertel-Blanc Study

Dr. Hans Hertel worked for many years as a food scientist with one of the major Swiss food companies that conducts business on a global scale. In 1991, he, along with Dr. Bernard Blanc of the University Institute for Biochemistry, conducted a quality clinical study to determine the effects of microwave cooking on food, and the resulting effects on the physiology of those who consumed the food.

The results of the study were sufficiently alarming such that in 1993, a powerful Swiss trade organization filed for, and obtained a "gag" order to prohibit publication of the findings. Finally, in 1998, a Swiss court determined that the gag order prohibiting Hertel from declaring that microwaved food is dangerous to health violated the right to freedom of expression. The order was reversed and the Swiss government was required to pay compensation.

Essentially, the Hertel-Blanc study found that microwave cooking significantly changes the food's nutrients, resulting in changes in the blood that could cause deterioration in the human body. More specifically, the study found a marked increase in the leukocytes in the blood. Leukocytes are of significant concern because they are often signs of pathogenic effects on living systems, such as poisoning and cell damage. The study also showed a decrease in white blood cells after consuming food cooked in a microwave oven.

The German and Russian Studies

William Koop has conducted an extensive review of the data from the German studies done in 1942-1943, and the Russian studies which began in 1957. His summary of the combined findings of the studies are presented here in three categories:

Effects on Nutritional Value of Food

Microwave exposure caused significant decreases in the nutritive value of all foods studied. The following are the most important findings to date:

Vitamins and In every food tested, the bioavailability of the
Minerals Made following vitamins decreased: vitamin B

Useless	complex, vitamins C and E, essential minerals and lipotropics.
Vital Energy Fields Devastated	The vital energy field content of all foods tested dropped 60 to 90%.
Digestibility of Fruits and Vegetables Reduced	Microwaving lowers the metabolic behavior and integration process capability of alkaloids, glucosides, lactosides and nitrolosides.
Meat Protein Worthless	It destroys the nutritive value of nucleoproteins in meats.
All Foods Damaged	It greatly accelerates the structural disintegration of all foods tested.

Cancer and Other Health Risks

The following effects have been observed when foods are subjected to microwave emissions:

Meats	Heating prepared meats sufficiently to insure sanitary ingestion created nitrosodiethanolamine, a well known cancer-causing agent.
Proteins	Active-protein, biomolecular compounds are destabilized.
Radioactivity	A "binding effect" between the microwaved food and any atmospheric radioactivity is created, causing a marked increase in the amount of alpha and beta particle saturation in the food.
Milk and Cereals	Cancer-causing agents are created in the protein-hydrolysate compounds of milk and cereal grains.
Frozen Foods	Microwaves used to thaw frozen foods alter the catabolism (breakdown) of the glucoside and

galactoside elements; both are glycosides (sugar derivatives) and found widely in plants.

Vegetables Even extremely brief exposure of raw, cooked or frozen vegetables to microwaves alters alkoloid catabolism, which can have a strong toxic effect on the human system.

Resulting Effects on the Human Body

Digestive System The unstable catabolism of microwaved foods alters their elemental food substances, causing disorders in the digestive system.

Lymphatic System Due to chemical alterations within food substances, malfunctions occur in the lymphatic system, causing a degeneration of the body's ability to protect itself against certain forms of neoplastics (cancerous growths).

Blood A higher-than-normal percentage of cancerous cells in blood serum (cytomas) can be seen in subjects ingesting microwaved foods.

Brain Their residual magnetism effect can render the psychoneural-receptor components of the brain more subject to influence by artificially induced, microwave radio frequency fields from transmission stations and TV relay networks.

Free Radicals Certain trace mineral molecular formations in plant substances (in particular, raw-root vegetables) form cancer-causing free radicals.

Stomach and Intestinal Cancers A statistically higher percentage of cancerous growths result in these organs, plus a generalized breakdown of the peripheral cellular tissues and a gradual degeneration of digestive and excretory functions.

Summary

Microwave ovens are found in more than 90% of the kitchens in the United States. Virtually every package of frozen or processed food that needs to be heated has instructions for microwave use. Even though there are growing concerns over the increasing incidence of cancer across a wide spectrum of the population, and a proliferation of health-related issues in young people, there has been an alarming void in microwave research conducted in this country. In view of the data from other countries, this void seems more than irresponsible.

Obviously, it is up to each of us to make our own decisions about the use of microwave ovens for cooking our daily meals. Perhaps we can blame the Nazis for inventing microwave ovens, but we can only blame ourselves if we continue to use them in light of the potential risks. Some health conscious people who have decided to discontinue using them for cooking have found a creative use for them – unplug them and use them as a place for storing your vegetarian cookbooks or for growing health-enhancing sprouts!

Chapter 18

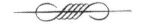

Food Irradiation

Although food irradiation has a different purpose and utilizes different technology than microwave ovens, many of the issues related to human health are similar.

What is food irradiation, and why is it used?

Let's start with the first part of the question. The nature of electromagnetic energy is characterized by its frequency of oscillation. Electromagnetic energy that is used for microwave ovens is in the range of about 2.4 trillion cycles per second, more commonly designated as 2.4 gigahertz, or abbreviated as 2.4 GHz. Electromagnetic waves in this frequency range cause molecules to move, but they cannot structurally change the atoms in those molecules.

On the other hand, electromagnetic energy that is used to irradiate food is at a much, much higher frequency – a frequency range that is commonly designated as X-ray, or the slightly higher frequency band referred to as gamma-rays. At these frequencies, the energies are capable of changing atoms by knocking an electron from them to form an ion. This form of energy radiation is known as ionizing radiation. But, energy in these frequency bands is not sufficiently intense to actual split atoms, causing objects exposed to this radiation to become radioactive. However, the potential danger is underscored by the fact that facilities using gamma sources for food irradiation must be licensed by the U.S. Nuclear Regulatory Commission.

Moving to the second half of the question, there are two primary purposes for food irradiation:

- Increasing the "shelf life" of foods, both before and after they are purchased by consumers. For example, irradiated strawberries stay unspoiled in a refrigerator for up to 3 weeks, as compared to 3 or 4 days for untreated berries.
- Reducing food-borne bacteria, viruses and parasites, such as Salmonella, E. coli, Campylobacter, Calicivirus (Norwalk-like viruses), Clostridium botulinum and Staphylococcus aureus.

The amount of ionizing radiation energy absorbed by a food item is measured in units called "kiloGrays," abbreviated as "kGy." Low doses, less than one kGy, inhibit the sprouting of tubers, such as potatoes, delay the ripening of some fruits and vegetables, control insects in fruits and stored grains, and reduce the problems of parasites in products of animal origin. Medium doses, 1-10 kGy, control pathogenic microbes responsible for food-borne illnesses and extend the shelf life of refrigerated foods. High doses, greater than 10 kGy, are not yet being commercially used for foods other than spices and dried vegetable seasonings, which are permitted to be irradiated up to 30 kGy.

Prior to 1985, the only foods approved for irradiation were spices, wheat, wheat flour and potatoes. Since then, there has been a progression of regulatory changes that have gradually, but dramatically, increased the array of foods that are permitted to be irradiated.

A major milestone was reached with the approval by the FDA in 1997, and the USDA in 1999, of irradiation for fresh and frozen red meats, such as beef, lamb and pork. The irradiation of poultry products had already been approved in 1992. On an international level, food irradiation has been approved in 41 different countries for up to 30 different food products.

In the United States, proponents of irradiation for controlling food-borne illnesses cite statistics from the Center for Disease

Control and Prevention which estimate that each year 76 million illnesses, 325,000 hospitalizations and 5,000 deaths occur due to food-borne illnesses. But others are concerned that if reliance is placed primarily on irradiation as a solution to this problem, sanitation standards in the food processing industry will gradually deteriorate. This concern is especially acute related to meat processing.

Health Concerns

There are three primary health concerns related to the irradiation of food:

- Does irradiation destroy most, if not all of the nutritional value of the food?
- Does irradiation create mutants and other agents in foods that result in carcinogens or other substances that impair human health?
- Have safety issues related to employees working in irradiation plants been adequately addressed?

Throughout the years, numerous studies have been done, primarily on laboratory animals, related to the ingestion of food that has been irradiated. Not surprisingly, the results are very disturbing. Following are a few examples based on a review of data from tests sponsored by the FDA and the U.S. Army Surgeon General:

- In a study of dogs, there was a 32% decrease in the surviving progeny of the dogs. The dogs on an irradiated food diet weighed 11.3% less than those in the control group. And, a significant number of carcinomas of the pituitary gland were found, an extremely rare type of malignant tumor.
- A 1968 FDA report indicated that a significant number of rats consuming irradiated beef died from internal

109

hemorrhage within 46 days, the first death coming after only 11 days.

- In 1959, the *Journal of Nutrition* reported on a study sponsored by the U.S. Army Surgeon General. In this case, rats fed irradiated beef all died within 34 days, again as a result of internal hemorrhaging.
- A 1960 study by the U.S. Army involved the feeding of the mice for two months before mating with half of the complete diet irradiated with gamma rays. This provoked a significant increase in embryonal deaths.
- In yet another study on rats reported in *Science* in 1963, a considerable number of second-generation rats in the experimental group that ate irradiated beef died. The rats most severely affected often became completely prostrated a short time before death. In no case were these symptoms observed in the control group. The possibility is that the afflicted ones were suffering from the characteristic muscular dystrophy syndrome referred to as nutritional muscular dystrophy, known to result from marginal vitamin E intake.
- Lastly, the *International Journal of Radiation Biology* cited a 1970 study of rats that were fed irradiated sucrose solutions. Considerable amounts of radioactivity were present in the liver, kidneys, stomach, gastrointestinal tract and blood serum of these rats. Radioactivity was also present in their urine and feces samples.
- A bulletin from the World Health Organization in 1969 stated: "Numerous studies have been carried out to ascertain whether cytotoxic effects occur when unirradiated biological test systems are cultured or fed with irradiated media or food. In such studies, adverse physiological growth retardation and inhibition, cytological cell division inhibition, chromosome aberrations and genetic effects have been observed in a wide range of test systems, ranging from bacteriophages to human cells. The available data

suggest that a variety of free radicals may act as the toxic and mutagenic agents."

Labeling of Irradiated Foods

The FDA currently requires that irradiated foods be labeled with a statement such as "treated with radiation" or "treated by irradiation." They must also display the international symbol for irradiation called the "radura," as shown at left. Foods labeled "organic" may not be radiated.

This labeling requirement does not apply to restaurants or other businesses that prepare and serve food. Therefore, there is no way to know whether or not you are eating irradiated food when dining out.

There are other significant flaws in the labeling requirements. Food products that contain food components that have been irradiated do not have to be labeled "irradiated." For example, foods that contain spices that have been irradiated with as much as 30kGy (the highest level of any food) do not have to be labeled as irradiated foods. In Canada, irradiated food components cannot constitute more than 10% of the total food product, otherwise they must be labeled as irradiated. In the United States, the FDA has caved in to pressure from the food conglomerates and modified the original legislation to allow food companies to have the irradiation warning labels in small print – as small as the labels that display the ingredients, and we all know how small that print usually is!

There also has been an attempt within the food industry to substitute the term "cold pasteurized" or even just "pasteurized" as a substitute for the irradiation labeling requirement. The 2002 Farm Bill authorizes potential use of the term "pasteurized" on any product that has been subjected to a significant pathogen reduction procedure of any type and allows companies to petition the FDA for the approval of using alternative labeling terms on irradiated food. The U.S. Department of Agriculture (USDA) awaits the FDA's decision on alternative labeling, and in the meantime considers the use of pasteurized labels on irradiated meat to be unacceptable.

Part 3

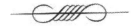

Balanced Lifestyle

Lifestyle is at least as important to our health as internal hygiene and nutrition. We all know the importance of exercise – some people get sufficient exercise in the course of their daily jobs, but most of us with a more sedentary lifestyle need to incorporate additional exercise in order to maintain a healthy body.

Adequate rest and sleep are also crucial factors. We may be able to go for short periods of time with minimal sleep, but in the long run, we simply cannot sustain our health on a diet of inadequate or irregular sleep habits.

The negative effects of smoking on our health have received so much attention during the past decade that there is no need to dwell on these in this book. It is clear by now that the detrimental effects of smoking are caused not just from the tobacco, but also from a long litany of chemicals that are added to cigarettes which drug the body, creating addition. Simply stated, smoking and good health are incompatible.

Perhaps less obvious are the effects of our thoughts and emotions on our health. Stress, anger, resentment and frustration all interfere with the healthy functioning of our body's organs and systems. On the other hand, love, joy, happiness and creative expression all have a positive impact our health and well-being.

In the following chapters, we shall explore these subjects in more detail.

Chapter 19

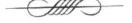

Exercise

Exercise is an essential part of a balanced lifestyle. In earlier times in a more agrarian culture, the daily activities involved in sustaining life provided most of the exercise that was needed to maintain a healthy body. However, as we have evolved into a more sedentary lifestyle, most of us need to consciously incorporate some form of additional exercise into our daily routines.

Some of the reasons why exercise is important are obvious; others less so. Following are some are some of the more important considerations:

Muscle Tone

Maintaining muscle tone and a physically attractive body is undoubtedly the most important motivator for most people when it comes to exercise. We know that muscles tend to atrophy if they are not regularly used. So for most of us, maintaining our muscles in good working condition and our body in good physical appearance is an important part of a healthy self-image.

Skeletal Mobility

The joints in our skeletal form need movement in order to maintain a full range of flexibility. The exercising we do to maintain muscle tone normally takes care of this need without special attention. However, certain types of stretching routines, such as yoga, can be very beneficial in maintaining an agile body.

Aerobic Exercises

Aerobic exercise uses large muscle groups in a rhythmic and continuous manner to elevate our heart rate and breathing for a sustained period of time. This can be in a simple form such as walking, jogging or swimming; or it can take a more rigorous form such as step, spin or dance routines found in many workout programs. Accelerated breathing that accompanies aerobic exercise brings more oxygen into the bloodstream. And the increased heart rate maximizes the flow of blood to all parts of the body.

Perspiration/Detoxification

The skin has an important role in eliminating toxins from the body through the sweat glands. So any exercise that causes a person to break into a sweat can be helpful in this regard. As the body generally becomes detoxified through the cleansing processes discussed in Part 1 of this book, and through an improved diet, the need for elimination of waste products through the sweat glands becomes less imperative.

Lymphatic System

The lymphatic system, which drains toxic and noxious substances from the connective tissues of the organs and muscles, depends on the daily movement of all the parts of the body to function properly. Unlike the blood, which has a heart to circulate it around the body, the lymph fluid has no such direct pumping device. The lymphatic system relies heavily on our breathing. When the muscle responsible for the breathing action of the lungs (diaphragm) extends into the abdomen, it exerts great pressure on the intestinal lymph vessels, thereby squeezing their contents. This forces the lymph to move through the lymph ducts. Thus, each inhalation and exhalation acts as an indirect pump for the lymphatic system. Shallow breathing that accompanies a sedentary lifestyle has a detrimental effect on proper lymph drainage. Exercise, however, can greatly improve lymphatic functions, thereby preventing a multitudes of diseases.

Cerebrospinal Fluid System

The cerebrospinal fluid circulates within the spinal column and the space between the inside of the skull and the surface of the brain. It is a primary conductor for life energies, or "chi", within the body. Like the lymphatic system, the cerebrospinal fluid system depends on the movement of the body, particularly deep breathing, to circulate its fluid.

Emotional Clearing

Emotions that cause tension, such as anger, fear or frustration, can become lodged in the muscular structure of the body. Regular physical exercise is an important aid to clearing these energies from the body before they create health problems.

Body-Mind-Spirit Integration

Some forms of exercise from Eastern traditions, such as Yoga, Tai Chi and Qigong, are designed to incorporate movement, breathing and mental focus in a way that promotes harmonious integration of body, mind and spirit. Ideally, they are done in a natural setting that can deepen our connection with the world of nature that surrounds us. But even if done in an indoor environment, they can provide needed exercise for our body in a way that nurtures all aspects of our beingness.

When and How Much?

The optimum type and amount of exercise naturally varies according to age, body type, and a variety of other factors. A 70 year old person does not need the same type or amount of exercise as a 20 year old.

- It is best not to exercise at more than 50% of your capacity, whatever that means to you. The purpose of exercising is not to prove to others how capable you are, but to derive personal benefit and satisfaction from it. If you are able to run for 30 minutes before you are tired, then make the choice to run only for 15 minutes. Getting tired during exercising defeats the very purpose of exercise. Feeling refreshed, revitalized and energetic afterwards indicates that the workout has been successful. In due time, your capacity for exercise will naturally increase on its own.

- Stop exercising when you feel the need to breathe through the mouth. Once you are forced to breathe through the mouth, rather than through the nose, you have gone beyond the 50% threshold of your capacity for exercise at that time. This is a sign that your body has moved into the adrenaline-breathing mode, which uses up your basic energy reserves and depletes cellular oxygen. You have reached your limit when you feel your heart pounding excessively, when you begin to sweat profusely, or when your body shakes. In that case it is good to finish off with a short period of walking and breathing normally. The basic rule is to always breathe through the nose and not through the mouth, and to exercise to the point of perspiration once a day.

- Additionally, it is best to exercise during daylight hours. Vigorous exercise in the evening hours is not healthy because the body needs to slow down to prepare itself for a restful and rejuvenating sleep. Never exercise just before or after a meal, as this interferes with the digestive process, and can cause indigestion. However, walking leisurely for 15 minutes after meals works as a good digestive aid. Always drink water before and after exercising to prevent the blood from thickening and the cells from becoming dehydrated.

Chapter 20

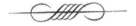

Daily Biological Cycles

The biological processes within our bodies are synchronized to the daily planetary cycles of light and darkness. By understanding the nature of these cycles, and adjusting our daily routines accordingly, we can better support our body's natural biological functions. The ancient science of Ayurveda divides the daily cycles into six 4-hour segments. Even though there are variations in the ratio of light to darkness as the Earth moves through its annual cycle around the Sun, the timing of the body's internal activities remains relatively consistent throughout the year.

6:00 AM to 10:00 AM

The first cycle begins with the "birth" of a new day. Let's assume that sunrise occurs at 6 am. About an hour before sunrise nature starts to awaken, becoming increasingly active as the sun rises to higher positions. Likewise, during this first segment of the day, your body is still a bit slow, but gradually gathers strength and stamina.

At around 6 am the kidney glands secrete the stress hormones cortisol and adrenaline to get your body going, similar to a battery starting an engine. This is also the time when the sex hormones in the body reach their peak levels. And, provided your eyes are open to see the natural light of the day, the brain increases its production of the powerful hormone serotonin, which helps you start your day on a positive note.

10:00 AM to 2:00 PM

By 10 am, the energy of the sun begins to increase, reaching its peak levels by about noon. During this 2-hour period, we are at our most alert and cognitive best. At noontime, the digestive energies reach their peak efficiency, and the digestive juices (bile, hydrochloric acid, enzymes, etc.) are profuse and concentrated. For this reason, it is best to eat your main meal of the day between 12 pm and 1 pm. Provided the food you eat is wholesome and nourishing, the digestive process will provide you with the energy and vitality you need during the remainder of the day.

2:00 PM to 6:00 PM

During this period, digestion of the noon meal continues. This segment of the day is conducive to efficient mental performance due to increased nerve cell activity. This makes it a good time to absorb and retain information. Studies conducted at the University of Wales showed that students who had afternoon or early-evening classes performed better in exams than those who had morning classes.

If there have been ongoing problems of poor intestinal absorption and unbalanced metabolism, they would likely become more pronounced at this time. Such an imbalance may manifest as increased irritability, nervousness and cravings for sugary foods or other stimulants such as tea, coffee, soft drinks, chocolate or cigarettes. Most alcoholics will start looking for their first drink during the latter part of this period.

6:00 PM to 10:00 PM

As the energies from the sun begin to fade, the physiological activities of the body such as digestion and metabolism begin to slow down. Those who are in tune with their body cycles usually feel inclined to take it easy with the arrival of the evening hours. For these reasons, it is best to eat only a light dinner, preferably at around 6 pm. This gives your body enough time to digest your food before bedtime. Research has found that the most important digestive enzymes are no longer produced after 8 pm. Eating a meal later in the evening (after 7 pm) will, therefore, not be properly digested and will decompose while it is still in the stomach.

Most people begin to feel sleepy or drowsy between 9 pm and 10 pm. This sleepiness or drowsiness results from the secretion of a natural tranquillizer that the brain makes when it wants you to go to sleep. According to researchers from Harvard Medical School, most of the brain cells are "turned off" during sleep by some chemical signal sent out by a group of cells located in the hypothalamus, which is considered to be the brain's brain. This "turning off the lights" assists us in going to sleep.

10:00 PM to 2:00 AM

This is a crucial period of time during which most of the body's energy is used for cleansing, rebuilding and rejuvenating the body. The liver receives most of the energy and conducts an astonishing range of activities. These include the supply of vital nutrients to all parts of the body, breaking down of noxious substances and keeping the blood clean. In addition, the liver cells produce bile at this time, which is needed to digest food, particularly fats, during the following day. Another important function of the liver during this time is to synthesize proteins, which serve as the main building blocks of cells, hormones and blood constituents.

Why Proper Sleep is So Important for You!

The liver requires all the energy it can get to fulfill these and many other responsibilities. This can only happen sufficiently, though, if you sleep during this time period. If you use up the nighttime energy for eating or for mental and physical activities, the liver is left with too little energy to do its extremely vital work. The kidneys also need energy during this time period to filter the blood plasma, and keep the body fluids balanced and blood pressure normal.

Although the brain makes up merely 2% of our body mass, it normally contains more than 25% of the body's entire blood supply. However, during this phase of the night, most of the blood located at the back of the brain moves into the liver for purification. If you are mentally or physically active at this time, the liver does not receive enough blood to work with, so it cannot cleanse the blood sufficiently. This results in the accumulation of toxic material in the blood stream. If toxins keep circulating in the blood, they will settle in the interstitial fluid (connective tissues) of organs and systems, thereby raising acidity and damaging them, including the liver itself. High blood toxicity can lead to secretions of stress hormones, brain fog, and injured capillaries, arteries and heart muscles. Most heart disease is the result of a poorly performing liver that is unable to remove all toxic, noxious substances from the blood on a daily basis. If we do not give the liver the energy it needs to conduct the most basic physiological activities, we sow the seeds of illness throughout the body.

Respiration is an important part of the cleansing and rejuvenation process, with a significant percentage of the body's waste materials being eliminated through the lungs.
This underscores the importance of sleeping in a room with ample ventilation.

Sleep can be divided into two main parts – before-midnight and after-midnight. For adults, the most important processes of purification and renewal occur during the two hours of sleep before midnight. This period involves deep sleep, often referred to as "beauty sleep." It typically lasts for about an hour, from 11 pm to midnight. During this period, you enter a dreamless state of sleep where oxygen consumption in the body drops considerably. This results in profound physical rest and relaxation. The benefit to your body of this single hour of deep sleep is approximately equivalent to that derived during the three hours following midnight, when the oxygen consumption rises again.

Growth factors, commonly known as growth hormones, are secreted profusely during the hour of deep sleep. These powerful hormones are responsible for cellular growth, repair and rejuvenation. People age faster if they don't produce enough growth hormones. The latest "fashion" in the beauty market is to consume synthetic growth hormones, which create remarkable rejuvenation results, but which also can have devastating side effects, including heart disease and cancer. On the other hand, if the body makes natural growth hormones at the right time and in the correct amounts, as happens during deep sleep, they can help keep the body vital and youthful.

Deep sleep virtually never occurs after midnight and it usually comes only if you go to sleep at least two hours before midnight. If you routinely miss out on deep sleep, your body and mind tend to become overtired. This triggers abnormal stress responses that initiate secretions of stress hormones such as adrenaline, cortisol or cholesterol (yes, cholesterol is a stress hormone that rises with stress!). Once the body's energy reserves have been depleted, chronic fatigue results. Fatigue can be considered a major contributing factor in today's health problems.

Doctors at the University of California at San Diego have found that losing a few hours of sleep not only makes you feel tired during the following day, but also can affect the immune system, possibly impairing the body's ability to fight infection. Since immunity diminishes with tiredness, your body is unable to defend itself against bacteria, microbes and viruses, and cannot cope with the build-up of harmful substances in the body.

2:00 AM to 6:00 AM

The primary focus of the body during this segment of the daily cycle is on moving the body's waste products from the liver, cells, intestines and other areas of the body towards the organs and systems of detoxification and elimination. The lymphatic system neutralizes harmful microbes, metabolic wastes, cellular debris, worn out cells and cells damaged by disease. The rectum forms fecal matter, which triggers a bowel movement, and the kidneys pass urine to the bladder, which induces urination. The skin also receives waste products that begin to surface at this time; hence, the importance of washing or showering in the morning.

To be able to fully support efficient waste removal, the body needs to be awake and in a vertical position. Therefore, it is preferable to awaken and be out of bed slightly before sunrise. Young children and early teenagers have a slightly different melatonin cycle, and may require an extra hour of sleep in the evening and again in the morning.

Summary

Structuring our daily lives in a way that honors our body's natural cycles is one of the most important things we can do to enhance our health and well-being. There are inevitably situations that arise in life that necessitate making exceptions to our normal daily cycle. But the more consistently we maintain a regular pattern of living, the better we are able to support our body's natural processes of health and regeneration.

Chapter 21

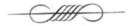

The Power of Our Thoughts and Emotions

In recent years there has been a growing awareness of how profoundly our health is affected by our thoughts and emotions. Hospitals have recorded innumerable cases generally known as "spontaneous remission," in which there has been a cessation of cancer or other serious illness soon after patients have changed the way they think and feel about themselves, or have shifted to a much more positive attitude toward life.[12]

The pioneering healing work of Louise Hay in assisting patients with AIDS has done much to highlight how by changing the way we think and feel about ourselves, we can bring about profound healing within our body. In her book, *You Can Heal Your Life*[7], she writes that the most common inner belief of the patients with whom she has worked is that they "are not good enough" or that they "don't deserve." She goes on to indicate that *resentment, criticism, guilt* and *fear* are the major causes of problems in our bodies and in our lives.

The human body has no built-in programs for sickness, but it has many programs to maintain a state of perfect balance. It is the nature of a human being to be healthy, but it is up to us to set the preconditions for these programs to work efficiently. Healing does not take place when there is no happiness. Bereaved persons, whose sense of joy has virtually become non-existent, demonstrate this most clearly. Widows rank among the highest in the risk groups for cancer. Sadness, due to the loss of a loved one, blocks a person's normal immune response to fight cancer cells, even though his or her T-cell count may be in the normal range. The latest studies on heart disease show that lack of happiness and job satisfaction head the list of risk factors for heart attacks.

In Bruce Lipton's recent book, *The Biology of Belief*,[11] he lays to rest the long-standing premise that it is our genes that control the biology of our body, and therefore our overall health. He describes how it is actually our thoughts and emotions that control our genes, which in turn carry out their important roles in the functioning of our bodies.

In 1989, Dr. Masaru Emoto,[6] of Japan, acquired a Magnetic Resonance Analyzer (MRA) to use in his medical practice. By analyzing certain energy patterns related to the specific illness to be treated, he was able to infuse related energy patterns into pure water, which his patients then drank. The use of this water, which he termed Hado water, yielded impressive healing results. However, many of his contemporaries in the scientific and medical communities remained skeptical. So, Dr. Emoto contemplated ways in which he might be able to display the energetic qualities that had been infused into the water.

One day he was reading an article about the crystalline structure of snowflakes, and was struck by the fact that no two snowflakes are identical. It occurred to him that since snowflakes are just frozen water, perhaps he could freeze Hado water, and then look at the ice crystals that were created. Success was not immediate, but through perseverance, he eventually was able to observe and photograph an incredibly beautiful water crystal.

As he continued his experiments, Dr. Emoto discovered that plain tap water from Tokyo would not produce such crystals. So he began to experiment with water from various sources, and found that pure water from natural sources such as springs or pristine streams and waterfalls consistently produces beautiful crystals of hexagonal form.

He eventually began to wonder if the nature of the ice crystals might be affected by thoughts, words or feelings projected into the water before freezing it. To his delight and amazement, he found that it made all the difference in the world! Through numerous experiments, Dr. Emoto found that the combination of the words "love" and "gratitude" seem to produce the most positive energy vibration, as reflected in the resultant crystals.

Considering that water accounts for approximately 65% of the body weight in humans, one can only imagine the extent to which we impact the health of our body by the thoughts we think and the words we speak.

It seems clear that the spiritual tradition of giving thanks and invoking a "blessing" on our food before we eat it is more than just of ceremonial significance. Remembering that "love" and "gratitude" combined create the most powerful crystalline-energetic structure, giving thanks for our food, and projecting "love" into it before we eat it, may not only energize the food in a positive manner, but also transform any impurities that may have been present in the food.

Chapter 22

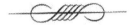

Our Body's Response to Stress

Stress is one of the greatest deterrents to health and well-being. Virtually all of us experience stress in our life from time to time, and our bodies are designed to respond accordingly. For example, if we encounter physical danger, the "fight or flight" stress responses within our body are designed to help us protect ourselves from that danger. So long as experiences of this nature are infrequent, our body is generally able to restore its normal equilibrium without any significant long-term effect on our health.

The more damaging situations are those to which we are exposed on a recurring basis, such as a stressful job, an inharmonious relationship or constant worries about finances. Even watching the daily television news programs tend to create levels of stress within us as we react emotionally to situations that seem tragic or unjust. Our book, *Lifting the Veil of Duality*,[(14)] addresses issues that tend to cause stress, and provides insights and guidance as to how we can live our life in peace and harmony even amid the seeming chaos of our contemporary world.

Growth or Protection

In his recently published book, *The Biology of Belief*,[(11)] Dr. Bruce Lipton discusses the concept of "growth or protection". Essentially this concept illustrates how the physiological processes within our body are dramatically affected by fear and stress.

The story begins at the cellular level. Dr. Lipton was a research biologist for many years; the focus of his work being on the functioning of human cells. One of the phenomena he noted early in his work was that if he placed human endothelial cells in the center of a culture dish, and then placed nutrients near the edge of the dish, the cells gradually migrated *toward* the nutrients. On the other hand, if he placed toxins near the edge of the dish, the cells would migrate *away* from the toxins. In other words, human cells would either move toward that which was nurturing, or away from that which was endangering. To say it another way, in any given moment, human cells are either in a state of "growth," or in a state of "protection."

Our human bodies are made up of approximately 50 trillion cells. Just like the individual cells, our bodies tend to be either in a state of growth or protection. The term "growth," as used here, is intended to imply not just growing in size from infancy to adulthood, but also the continual sustenance and regeneration of our bodies throughout our lifetime.

The growth center of our body is the "visceral" area, which includes the digestive system, and organs such as the lungs, heart, liver, and kidneys – all of the organs that play a key role in the sustenance and regeneration of our body. The protection aspect of our body involves two facets: *internal* protection and *external* protection. The primary system with responsibility for internal protection is the immune system. Our external protection involves the somatic system, such as our arms and legs that enable us to respond to a "fight or flight" situation.

Under normal circumstances, if our life situation is reasonably peaceful and we feel a sense of security, our body will be in a state of growth most of the time. However, if we are suddenly confronted with a dangerous situation, such as an earthquake, our body immediately shifts to a state of protection. This shift is initiated by our nervous system, working through our endocrine glands.

When our body shifts from a state of growth to a state of protection, we are impacted in three primary ways:

- The flow of blood is constricted in our visceral area, and re-directed to our somatic system (arms, legs, etc.). Consequently, the functioning of our life-sustaining

128

systems, such as our digestive system, is throttled back to a minimum.

- Since the threat in the example of an earthquake is an *external* threat, rather than an *internal* threat, the immune system is essentially put on temporary hold in order to conserve energy and make it available for somatic activity. This is analogous to the situation involving a modern commercial airplane – just prior to heading down the runway for takeoff, the pilot turns off auxiliary systems such as the air conditioner, so that all of the thrust of the engines is available to support lift-off.

- The blood flow in the brain is re-directed from the forebrain, where our rational thinking takes place, to the hindbrain, which involves our reflex responses. Since it is the frontal lobes of the forebrain that support rational thinking, when we shift into a state of protection, our ability to think logically is impaired. We frequently hear stories of experienced hikers that become lost in bad weather. If fear and panic overtake a hiker, they often do not make rational survival decisions. For example, they may continue to hike aimlessly as fast as they can to the point of exhaustion, rather than using their energy to build a shelter in which to wait out the storm.

If our body remains in a state of protection for a relatively short period of time, little damage is done to our internal growth-related processes. However, unlike each individual cell that at any point in time is either totally in a state of growth or state of protection, the collective of cells that constitute our body can exist in gradational states somewhere between total growth and total protection. This is the state in which we are likely to find ourselves if our life is regularly taxed under excessive stress.

For example, we know that under conditions of stress or turmoil, we frequently suffer from indigestion. We also know that during periods of stress, we are more likely to come down with a cold, or experience other aches and pains within our body. We may, or may not be aware that our rational mind does not function as well under stressful situation. Since it is our rational mind that is the "observer" of our thinking ability under such situations, the observer, itself, may not be able to observe clearly.

In his book, Dr. Lipton goes on to describe how this concept of "growth or protection" affects the development of a fetus during pregnancy. The evolving fetus lives in the emotional field of the mother, and is dramatically impacted in its development by these emotions. If the mother's emotions are normally peaceful and loving, then the forebrain of the fetus will develop in a normal, healthy manner. However, if the mother is frequently in a state of fear and anger, nature prepares the fetus to live in a correspondingly harsh emotional environment after birth. So it directs the hindbrain to be developed more fully, at the expense of the development of the forebrain. Dr. Lipton points out that the intelligence of a child can be affected by as much as 50%, depending on the emotional environment in which its development took place while in the womb.

Dr. Lipton's DVD/video[25] entitled "Nature, Nurture and the Power of Love" provides important information for all of us as to how our body is affected by our thoughts and emotions. It carries an especially important message for young couples that are thinking about starting a family.

Chapter 23

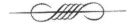

Living Consciously

To live *consciously* is to re-create our life the way we want it to be. Good health and vitality are our natural birthright. No matter what our age or our current health situation is, it is never too late to make positive changes that will help us heal ourselves, so that we may live life to the fullest.

We are constantly being bombarded with words and images through television, movies, magazines and other media that are designed to influence our life choices. Much of this is overt, such as cleverly conceived advertising created to appeal to a target group of individuals. Some is more subtle, designed to reinforce our cultural behaviors.

All of us are familiar with the barrage of commercials by the pharmaceutical industry promoting one drug or another as the solution for various health problems. Somewhat less obvious is that ever present reminder in these advertisements to "ask your doctor whether 'drug-x' is right for you," perpetuating the idea that your doctor is the ultimate authority when it comes to making health decisions in your life.

To live consciously means to take charge of our own life, including our health decisions. Yes, doctors have an important role in our health care system, especially in dealing with trauma such as physical injuries. But we need to better educate ourselves as to how our bodies function, and how we can work with the natural processes of our body to support health and vitality.

Making life decisions based on *inner wisdom*, rather than *outside influences*, represents a fundamental change for many people. It is not always easy to go against the cultural currents – to be the one that is always "different" when we are with a group of friends.

Changing our life begins with clarifying our intentions. Let's explore this in a bit more detail. Our intentions are literally a field of energy that we radiate out from the center of our being – our 'heart' center – as we move through the experiences of our daily life. This field of energy consists of both our thoughts and our emotions, integrated together in a unified field.

If upon waking in the morning, we take a few moments to clarify our intentions for the day, we literally pre-program the nature of the experiences that we will attract to us. For example, if we affirm that it is our intention to be kind to each person we meet, and if we take a few moments in our imagination to move into the *feelings* of what those encounters will be like, then we will proceed through our day radiating the energies of kindness. A resonance will occur as we encounter others who are also radiating an intention (unified energy field) of kindness. Through their "inner sense," or "intuition," they will be attracted to interact with us on the vibration of kindness. The interaction might be as simple as a smile as they pass by us, or something more expansive.

On the other hand, if we live unconsciously, and allow our intentions to be dominated by negative thoughts and emotions, there will be a resonance with others who are radiating similar negative thoughts and emotions. Consequently, our experiences throughout the day are likely to be of a much more negative or depleting nature, reinforcing our own negativity.

Relating this to personal wellness, if we begin our day by affirming our intention to do only those things throughout the day that contribute to our health and vitality, we will tend to live our life in a healthier manner. Making changes in our life is seldom easy or instantaneous. Nevertheless, like a child learning to walk, if we begin with small steps and pay attention to the progress we are making, we can develop the confidence that is needed to take larger steps.

In his book, *The Power of Intention: Learning to Co-Create Your World Your* Way,[5] Dr. Wayne Dyer writes about intention as being a field of energy that flows invisibly beyond the reach of our normal, everyday habit patterns. He goes on to say that this omnipresent power of intention pervades everything and everyone, so all we need to do to be what we want to be, and to achieve what we want to achieve is to align our intention, and then everything in the universe will assist us.

Living consciously involves the integration and alignment of our body, mind and spirit in a way that provides the courage and wisdom to make important life choices from within, rather than simply responding to external influences.

Chapter 24

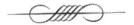

"The natural force within each one of us
is the greatest healer of disease."

Hippocrates

Conclusion

Living a life of health and vitality is our natural birthright. It has been our intent in this book to provide information about how each of us can work with the natural processes of our body to cleanse the accumulated residues from our various organs and systems, and to make wise choices about the foods we eat. We have also provided examples of how our health is impacted by our thoughts, emotions and lifestyle.

It is beyond the scope of this book to discuss various natural therapies such as body work, homeopathy, color therapy, acupuncture, essence therapy, and many others. But we want to acknowledge their value and importance in achieving and maintaining optimum health.

Although our focus has been on working with the natural processes of our bodies, we certainly do not want to imply that conventional Western medicine is of no value. It is difficult to imagine what our world would be like without emergency rooms to deal with trauma such as physical injuries.

Our hope is that through this book you will be inspired to learn more about how your body functions so that you will be able to make enlightened decisions related to your health and well-being. We invite you to take your health into your hands and feel empowered by the wealth of life-nurturing choices at your fingertips.

Appendix A

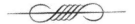

Applied Kinesiology: "Muscle Testing"

Everything that we experience physically, mentally or emotionally affects our entire being. For example, we may be feeling fine, happily going about our day, and then receive a phone call that informs us of the accidental death of a close friend. Immediately, everything shifts. On a physical level, we may start to feel weak and nauseous as we attempt to deal with the news we have just received.

On the other hand, if under the same circumstances the telephone message indicated that we had just become grandparents, and that baby and mother were doing just fine, we would most likely experience radiations of joy and gratitude throughout our body. In this euphoric state, our body would respond in an entirely different manner than in the previous example.

Applied Kinesiology involves the inter-relationships of our thoughts, emotions and body as we experience the world around us. Every substance radiates a vibration, or frequency. If we are in an environment that contains toxic substances, the radiations from those substances will affect us in a negative way. Similarly, if we are walking in the mountains through a field of wild flowers, the radiations from the flowers are likely to affect us in a positive manner.

Our subconscious mind controls our autonomic nervous system and is responsible for our automatic physical and neurological functions. For example, if we consciously decide to walk from our bedroom to the kitchen, our subconscious mind takes over and directs all of the appropriate muscles in our body to accomplish this task. It is also our subconscious mind that directs the myriad functions of the organs and systems of our body. In this sense, we may think of our subconscious mind as the "wisdom" of our body.

Our body wisdom knows from the radiations of any particular food whether or not that food will be healthy or unhealthy for our body at the present time. "Muscle testing" is an application of kinesiology. It enables us to use the wisdom of our body to test various food substances to determine whether or not they are healthy for us. Rather than attempting to understand the neurological-physiological science involved in this process, we recommend that you simply experience the process for yourself, and see if it works for you.

Muscle Testing Procedure

Although there are muscle testing procedures that can be done alone, the procedure we recommend, at least as a starting point, requires a partner.

Step 1

Face your partner as illustrated in Figure 1. The person being tested extends one of their arms out parallel to the floor. Either arm can be used, but it is best not to use an arm that is sore or injured. The tester lightly grasps (between their thumb and four fingers) the wrist of the extended arm. The tester's other arm should rest lightly on the shoulder of the outstretched arm for stability. The person being tested keeps their body relaxed, their head upright, but with their eyes open and looking downward toward the floor. Be sure this person does not tip the head forward.

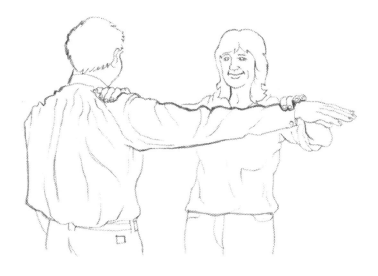

Figure 1

Step 2

This step involves establishing kinesthetic communication between the person doing the testing and the person being tested. To begin, have the person being tested think of something that makes them feel very good, such as a dear friend or a delightful experience. When the person being tested is ready, the tester should say "be strong," and then immediately apply some downward pressure on the wrist. The person being tested should resist the downward pressure, and attempt to keep their arm parallel to the floor. This will provide both the tester and the person being tested an opportunity to sense how strong the arm is when positive thoughts are being held in their mind.

Step 3

Next, have the person being tested think of something or someone they don't like. As in Step 2, when ready the tester should say "be strong," and again apply downward pressure on the wrist. This time the person being tested is likely to have more difficulty resisting the downward pressure, with the extended arm ending up in the position illustrated in Figure 2.

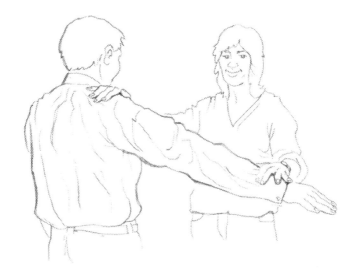

Figure 2

Step 4

Practice this process a few times to get the feel of it. When the tester applies downward pressure, it should be in moderation. The purpose is not to see who is stronger, but rather to mutually gain a sense as to when the arm is stronger or when it is weaker. The reason for saying "be strong" just before applying the downward pressure is that it alerts the person being tested to resist the downward pressure that will be coming momentarily. If the arm gets tired, either switch arms, or just rest for a short while.

You might want to experiment to become more comfortable with the testing process. For example, instead of thinking of something that makes you feel good, you might want to make a statement that you know is true. You might say something like "ice is cold." The outstretched arm should then test strong. And instead of thinking of a person or situation that you don't like, you may want to say something that you know is false, like "ice is hot." The arm should then test weak.

Step 5

You are now ready to start testing food substances. You might want to start with a container of white sugar. With one arm outstretched as before, hold the sugar in your other hand. While holding the sugar, make a statement such as "this sugar is healthy for me." Then, as before, the tester says "be strong," and immediately applies downward pressure on the outstretched arm. In this case, the arm is likely to be weak, and drop to the position illustrated in Figure 2.

Next, select another food sample, perhaps a clump of broccoli, and repeat the testing process. By testing several different food samples, you will probably be able to determine the effect each one has on the strength of your arm – the healthier a particular food is for you, the stronger your arm will be. Likewise, the less healthy a food is for you, the weaker your arm will be. If you find your arm getting tired, be sure to switch arms or stop and rest for a while, otherwise the testing will not be accurate.

Summary

The wisdom of your body does not lie.[4] If you are performing the tests properly, the results should be reliable. With additional practice you will probably learn not only to determine if a food item is healthy or unhealthy for you, but also the degree to which it is beneficial or detrimental.

There are other techniques available to tap into the wisdom of the body, such as the use of a pendulum or energy wand. You might want to try various methods to see which one works best for you. One advantage of a pendulum or energy wand is that it does not require a partner.

Appendix B

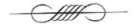

The Kidney Cleanse

If the presence of gallstones in the liver or other factors have led to the occurrence of sand or stones in the kidneys or the urinary bladder, you may also need to cleanse the kidneys.

The kidneys are very delicate, blood-filtering organs that easily get congested through poor digestion, stress and an irregular lifestyle. The main causes of congestion in the kidneys are kidney stones. Most kidney crystals/stones, however, are too small to be recognized through modern diagnostic instruments, such as X-ray.

The following herbs, when taken daily for a period of 20-30 days, can help dissolve and eliminate all the various types of kidney stones, including uric acid stones, oxalic acid stones, phosphate stones and amino acid stones. If you have a history of kidney stones, in order to completely clean out your kidneys you may need to repeat this cleanse several times, at intervals of 6-8 weeks.

Ingredients

1. Marjoram (1oz.)
2. Cat's Claw (1oz.)
3. Comfrey Root (1oz.)
4. Fennel Seed (2oz.)
5. Chicory Herb (2oz.)
6. Uva Ursi (2oz.)
7. Hydrangea Root (2oz.)
8. Gravel Root (2oz.)
9. Marshmallow Root (2oz.)
10. Golden Rod Herb (2oz.)

Note: An herbal store in Minneapolis, Minnesota, The Present Moment Book & Herbs, has these herbs available already mixed together in the proper proportions. See the "Sources" page in the back of this book for more information.

Directions

Take 1 oz. each of the first three herbs and 2 oz. each of the rest of the herbs and thoroughly mix them together. Keep them in an airtight container. Before bedtime, soak 2-3 heaping tablespoons of the mixture in two cups of water, cover it and leave covered overnight.

The next morning, bring the concoction to a boil. Let it simmer for a few minutes and then strain it. If you forget to prepare the tea in the evening, bring it to a boil in the morning and let it lightly simmer 10-15 minutes before straining.

Drink a few sips at a time in 6-8 intervals throughout the day. This tea does not have to be taken warm or hot, but do not refrigerate it. Do not add sugar or sweeteners. Leave at least one hour after eating before taking your next sips.

Repeat this procedure for 20-30 days. If you experience discomfort or stiffness in the lower back area during the cleanse, it is because salt crystals from kidney stones are passing through the ureter ducts of the urinary system. Any strong smell or darkening of the urine at the beginning or middle of the cleanse indicates a major release of toxins from the kidneys. Usually, the release is gradual and does not significantly change the color or texture of the urine.

Important: During the cleanse, support the kidneys by drinking extra amounts of water, a minimum of 6 and a maximum of 8 glasses per day.

During the cleanse, avoid consuming animal products, dairy foods, tea, coffee, alcohol, carbonated beverages, chocolate and any other foods or beverages that contain preservatives, artificial sweeteners or coloring agents. While cleansing the kidneys, harsh substances such as chemicals may not only interfere with the cleanse, but may also injure the kidneys.

In addition to drinking this kidney tea each day, you may chew a small piece of rind from an organic lemon on the left side of your mouth and a small piece of carrot on the right side of your mouth, 30-40 times each. This stimulates the kidney functions. Make certain that there is at least half an hour in between chewing 'cycles.'

A Cautionary Note: If you are over 70 or quite sick, do the kidney cleanse for six weeks. If you have a history of kidney stones, or have been diagnosed as having large kidney or bladder stones, or have chronic pain or stiffness in the loin areas, toes or fingers, you may need to add the following alkalization procedure to the kidney cleanse:

1. Check the acidity of your urine with a pH-indicator, a special paper used for measuring urinary pH, available at most drugstores. First thing in the morning, hold a small piece of this paper in the urine stream. If it indicates a pH of 5.5 or below, the acidity level may be too high, indicating that you require an alkalizing treatment. You should have a morning urine pH of about 6. Most people with painful joints have a morning urine pH of about 4.5, which means that more uric acid is precipitated during the night. This can cause severe pain in the morning hours. During the day, the urinary pH tends to be less acidic and sufferers tend to feel better as some of the acid deposits are neutralized.

2. To alkalize the body, mix two parts *sodium bicarbonate* (baking soda) and one part *sodium potassium* in a glass jar. Put one level teaspoon of this mixture in one large glass of water (not cold) and drink it at bedtime, at least 2 hours after dinner. If possible, drink it all at once. The next morning your urine pH should be at about 6. If not, increase the dose to one heaping teaspoon. Check your pH from time to time, as you may need to reduce the dose, to maintain a pH of 6. By alkalizing yourself at bedtime, you prevent the urinary pH from dropping too low during the night. This will reduce the deposits in the joints and, at the same time, prevent dissolved kidney crystals from reassembling themselves into new

stones. Continue this alkalizing procedure throughout the kidney cleanse or as long as there is pain in your toes or fingers.

Note: If sodium potassium is not available, use only sodium bicarbonate. The dosage should be one-half teaspoon (or more if needed) in a glass of water at bedtime.

Appendix C

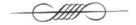

List of Alkaline-forming and Acid-forming Foods

Following is a list of common foods and beverages, showing the degree to which they are alkaline-forming or acid-forming.[2] Fruits and vegetables are categorized based on their natural state. Any process such as cooking, freezing, canning or preserving with sugars and chemicals greatly reduces the alkaline-forming qualities; in many cases transforming them into acid-forming foods.

Fruits & Berries

Extremely
Alkaline-forming:

Cantaloupe
Dates (dried)
Figs (dried)
Lemons
Limes
Mangos
Melons (all
varieties)
Papaya
Watermelon

Moderately
Alkaline-forming:
Apples
Apricots

Bananas (ripe)
Citron
Currants
Gooseberries
Grapes (sweet
varieties)
Grapefruit
Guavas
Kiwis
Kumquats
Passion Fruit
Peaches
Pears
Persimmons
Pineapple
Quince
Raisins
Tangerines

Slightly Alkaline-
forming:

Carob (powdered
pod)
Cherries
Grapes (sour
varieties)
Oranges
Pomegranate
Raspberries
Strawberries

Slightly Acid-
forming:

Blueberries
Cranberries

145

Plums   Prunes

Grains

Note: Acid-forming grains become slightly alkaline-forming when sprouted.

Slightly Alkaline-forming:

Amaranth
Millet
Quinoa

Slightly Acid-forming:
Barley
Corn meal
Rye
Spelt

Moderately Acid-forming:

Basmati rice
Brown rice
Buckwheat
Oats
Wheat (whole)

Extremely Acid-forming:

Wheat (bleached)
White rice

Vegetables & Herbs

Extremely Alkaline-forming:

Kelp
Parsley
Seaweed (all types)
Watercress

Moderately Alkaline-forming:

Asparagus
Carrots
Celery
Chard (Swiss)
Dandelion greens
Endive
Lettuce (leaf)

Potatoes (with peel)
Pumpkin
Rutabaga
Spinach
Squash (varies slightly by type)

Mildly Alkaline-forming:

Artichokes (Jerusalem)
Bamboo shoots
Beets
Broccoli
Brussels sprouts
Cabbage
Cauliflower
Chicory

Collard greens
Corn (sweet)
Cucumber
Eggplant
Ginger (fresh)
Kale
Kohlrabi
Leeks
Mustard greens
Okra

Onion
Parsnip
Pepper (Bell)
Potato
Radish
Swiss chard
Tomato
Turnip
Water chestnut

Beans

Note: Acid-forming beans become alkaline-forming when sprouted.

Moderately Alkaline-forming:

Green (fresh)
Lima (fresh)
Peas (fresh)
Snap (fresh)
String (fresh)

Slightly Alkaline-forming:

Soybeans (and soybean
products)

Slightly Acid-forming:

Aduki
Black
Garbanzo
Kidney
Lentils
Mung
Navy
Pinto
Red
White

Nuts

Note: Cooking, smoking or roasting nuts reduces the alkaline-forming quality, and makes acid-forming more extreme. It also destroys certain vitamins, making them harder to digest. Soaking nuts in water overnight increases their alkaline-forming quality. It also eliminates the anti-digestive enzyme normally found in nuts, and is therefore the preferred way to prepare them for ingestion.

Pignolias

Slightly Acid-forming:
Brazil

Moderately Alkaline-forming:
Cashew
Coconut (dried)

Almonds (powerful anti-cancer
food)
Filbert (hazelnut)
Macadamia
Coconut (fresh)
Peanut
Pecan
Slightly Alkaline-forming:
Pistachio
Chestnuts (dry roasted)
Walnut

Seeds

Note: Most sprouted seeds are moderately alkaline-forming. Unsprouted seeds (with the exception of sesame) are acidic. The high content of utilizable organic calcium places sesame in a special category.

Moderate Alkaline-forming:

Slightly Acid-forming:
Alfalfa (sprouted)
Chia (sprouted)
Pumpkin
Radish (sprouted)
Sunflower
Sesame (unsprouted)

Meats

Moderately Acid-forming:

Extremely Acid-forming:

Fish
Red meat
Shellfish
Poultry

Beverages

Alkaline-forming:

Fresh fruit and vegetable juices
   (The same as the fruits and
   vegetables from which
derived.)

Moderately Alkaline-forming:

Herbal Teas:
     Alfalfa (leaf)
     Clover (leaf)
     Mint (leaf)
     Sage (leaf)
     Spearmint (leaf)

Slightly Alkaline-forming:

Herbal Teas:
     Raspberry (leaf)
     Strawberry (leaf)
     Comfrey (leaf or root)
     Ginseng (leaf or root))
     Ginger (root)

Extremely Acid-forming:

Alcoholic drinks (liquor, wine,
beer)
Coffee
Soft drinks
Black tea

Processed Foods

Virtually all processed foods are moderately to extremely acid-forming. This includes pasta, pastries and baked foods – especially those made with refined flours.

Appendix D

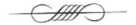

Acid Symptom Checklist

Following is a list of symptoms that commonly result from an excess of acidic residues in the cells and tissues throughout the body.[2]

BEGINNING SYMPTOMS

Acne
Agitation
Muscular pain
Cold hands and feet
Dizziness
Low energy
Joint pains that travel
Food allergies
Chemical sensitivities to odors,
gas heat
Hyperactivity
Panic attacks
Pre-menstrual and menstrual
cramping
Pre-menstrual anxiety and
depression

Lack of sex drive; weak libido
Bloating
Heartburn
Diarrhea
Constipation
Hot urine
Strong smelling urine
Mild headaches
Rapid panting breath
Rapid heartbeat
Irregular heartbeat
White coated tongue
Hard to get up in morning
Excess head mucous (stuffiness)
Metallic taste in mouth

INTERMEDIATE SYMPTOMS

Cold sores (Herpes I & II)
Depression
Loss of memory
Loss of concentration
Migraine headaches

Insomnia
Disturbance in smell, taste,
vision, hearing
Asthma
Bronchitis

Hay fever
Ear aches
Hives
Swelling
Viral infections (colds, flu)
Bacterial infections (staph, strep)
Fungal infections (candida albicans, athelete's foot, vaginal yeast infection)
Impotence

Urethritis
Cystitis
Urinary infection
Gastritis
Colitis
Excessive falling hair
Psoriasis
Endometriosis
Stuttering
Numbness and tingling
Sinusitis

ADVANCED SYMPTOMS

Crohn's Disease
Schizophrenia
Learning disabled
Hodgkin's Disease
Systemic Lupus Erythematosis
Multiple Sclerosis
Sarcoidosis

Rheumatoid Arthritis
Myasthenia Gravis
Scleroderma
Tuberculosis
Leukemia
All other forms of cancer

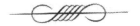

Food Groups

Protein

Meat (red)
Fish
Seafood
Poultry
Wild game
Milk

Cheese
Yogurt
Beans
Peas

Cereals
Seeds
Nuts
Legumes
Peanuts

Starch

Grains
Pastas
Rice
Corn
Potato (all)

Turnip
Squash
Pumpkin
Parsnip
Beet

Carrot
Eggplant
Avocado

"Green" Vegetables

Asparagus
Artichoke
Beans (green)
Broccoli
Brussels sprouts
Cabbage
Cauliflower
Celery
Chives
Collard greens
Cucumber

Dandelion greens
Endive
Eggplant
Garlic
Kale
Kohlrabi
Leeks
Lettuce
Okra
Onion

Parsley
Peppers (all)
Radish
Rhubarb
Scallion
Sea vegetables
Spinach
Swiss chard
Turnip
Watercress
Zucchini

Fruits (sweet)

Banana	Raisin	Prune
Date	Grape (sweet)	Pear (sun-dried)
Fig	Persimmon	

Fruits (Sub-Acid)

Apple (sweet)	Huckleberry	Pear
Apricot	Mango	Papaya
Cherry (sweet)	Peach (sweet)	Plum

Fruits (Acid)

Apple (sour)	Pineapple	Lemon
Orange	Pomegranate	Lime
Grapefruit	Tomato	

Melons

Cantaloupe	Crenshaw	Musk
Casaba	Honeydew	Watermelon

References

Books and Reports

1. Batmanghelidj, Fereydoon, MD. *Your Body's Many Cries for Water*. Global Health Soultions, Inc., Falls Church, NC, 1992.

2. Baroody, Theodore A., ND, DC, Ph.D. *Alkalize or Die*. Holographic Health Press, Waynesville, NC, 1991.

3. Blauer, Stephen. *The Juicing Book*. Avery, Penguin Group, Inc. USA, 1989.

4. Diamond, John. *Your Body Doesn't Lie*. Warner Books, New York, NY, 1979.

5. Dyer, Wayne, Ph.D. *The Power of Intention: Learning to Create Your World Your Way*. Hay House, Inc., Carlsbad, CA, 2004.

6. Emoto, Masaru. *Hidden Messages in Water*. (Translated by David A. Thayne). Beyond Words Publishing, Inc., Hillsboro, OR 2004.

7. Hay, Louise L. *You Can Heal Your Life*. Hay House, Inc., Carlsbad, CA, 1984.

8. Jensen, Bernard, DC, Ph.D. *Guide to Body Chemistry and Nutrition*. Keats Publishing, Los Angeles, CA, 2000.

9. Jensen, Bernard, DC, Ph.D. *Foods that Heal*. Avery, Penguin Group, Inc. USA, 1988.

10. Jensen, Bernard, DC, Ph.D. *The Healing Power of Chlorophyll from Plant Life*. Bernard Jensen Enterprises, Escondido, CA 1973.

11. Lipton, Bruce H., Ph.D. *The Biology of Belief.* Mountain of Love/Elite Books, Santa Rosa, CA, 2005.

12. Moritz, Andreas. *Cancer Is Not A Disease: It's A Survival Mechanism.* Ener-Chi Press, Greenville, SC, 2005.

13. Moritz, Andreas. *It's Time to Come Alive.* Ener-Chi Press, Greenville, SC, 1998.

14. Moritz, Andreas. *Lifting the Veil of Duality.* Ener-Chi Press, Greenville, SC, 2001.

15. Moritz, Andreas. *Timeless Secrets of Health and Rejuvenation.* Ener-Chi Press, Greenville, SC, 1997.

16. Moritz, Andreas. *The Amazing Liver and Gallbladder Flush.* Ener-Chi Press, Greenville, SC, 1998.

17. Null, Gary, Ph.D.; Carolyn Dean, MD, ND; Martin Feldman, MD; Debora Rasio, MD, Dorothy Smith, Ph.D. *Death by Medicine.* December 2003.

18. Oski, Frank A. , MD. *Don't Drink Your Milk.* TEACH Services, Inc., Brushton, NY, 1996.

19. Robbins, John. *Diet For A New America.* H. K. Kramer, Tiburon, CA 1987.

20. Shelton, Herbert M. *Food Combining Made Easy.* Dr. Shelton's Health School, San Antonio, TX 1951.

21. Vasey, Christopher, ND. *The Acid-Alkaline Diet for Optimum Health.* (Translated by Jon Graham). Healing Arts Press, Rochester, VT, 2003.

22. Walker, N. W. *Raw Vegetable Juices: What's Missing in Your Body?* Norwalk Press, Phoenix, AZ, 1970.

23. Whang, Sang. *Reverse Aging.* JSP Publishing, Miami, FL 1990.

24. Wigmore, Ann. *The Wheatgrass Book.* Avery, Penguin Group, Inc. USA, 1985.

DVD/Videos

25. Lipton, Bruce H., Ph.D. *Nature, Nurture and the Power of Love.* Mountain or Love Productions, www.brucelipton.com.

Sources

Herbs for Kidney Cleanse

The Present Moment
3546 Grand Avenue
Minneapolis, MN 55408
USA
Order by Telephone:
800-378-3245
612-824-3157
E-mail: herbshop@presentmoment.com
Website: www.presentmoment.com

Colema Board Colon Cleanse Equipment

Colema Board of California, Inc.
3660 Main Street, Suite C
Cottonwood, CA 96022
Telephone: 800-745-2446

Ionic Water-soluble Minerals

ENIVA Corporation
P.O. Box 49755
Minneapolis, MN 55449
U.S.A.
Toll Free: 1-866-999-9191
Tel: 1-763-398-0005
Fax: 1-763-795-8890
Web Site: http://www.eniva.com
Note: To order any products from Eniva, you require a sponsor name
and ID. You may use the name and ID of the author, Andreas Moritz,
#13462. Or order direct from this we site:
https://www.enivamembers.com/enerchi

Books by Andreas Moritz
Ener-Chi Wellness Center
E-mail: EnerChiArt@aol.com
Website: www.ener-chi.com

DVD/Video by Bruce Lipton
Websites: www.brucelipton.com
          www.spirit2000.com
Telephone: 800-550-5571

ABOUT THE AUTHORS

Andreas Moritz

Andreas Moritz is a medical intuitive, a practitioner of Ayurveda, Iridology, Shiatsu and Vibrational Medicine, a writer and artist. Born in Southwest Germany in 1954, Andreas had to deal with several severe illnesses from an early age, which compelled him to study diet, nutrition and various methods of natural healing while still a child.

By the age of 20, Andreas had completed his training in Iridology – the diagnostic science of eye interpretation – and Dietetics. In 1981, he began studying Ayurvedic Medicine in India and completed his training as a qualified practitioner of Ayurveda in New Zealand in 1991. Rather than being satisfied with merely treating the symptoms of illness, Andreas has dedicated his life's work to understanding and treating the root causes of illness. Because of this holistic approach, he has had astounding success with cases of terminal disease where conventional methods of healing proved futile.

Since 1988, he has been practicing the Japanese healing art of Shiatsu, which has given him profound insights into the energy system of the body. In addition, he devoted eight years of active research into consciousness and its important role in the field of mind/body medicine.

Andreas Moritz is the author of *The Amazing Liver & Gallbladder Flush, Timeless Secrets of Health and Rejuvenation, Lifting the Veil of Duality, Cancer is Not a Disease, It's Time to Come Alive,* and *The Art of Self-Healing* (mid-2006).

During his extensive travels throughout the world, he has consulted with heads of state and members of government in Europe, Asia, and Africa, and has lectured widely on the subject of health, mind/body medicine and spirituality. His popular *Timeless Secrets of Health and Rejuvenation* workshops assist people in taking responsibility for their own health and well-being. Andreas runs a free forum "Ask Andreas Moritz" on the popular health website Curezone.com (5 million readers and increasing).

After taking up residency in the United States in 1998, Andreas has been involved in developing a new innovative system of healing – *Ener-Chi Art* – which targets the root causes of many chronic illnesses. Ener-Chi Art consists of a series of light ray-encoded oil paintings that can instantly restore vital energy flow (Chi) in the organs and systems of the body.

Andreas is also the founder of *Sacred Santèmony – Divine Chanting for Every Occasion,* a powerful system of specially generated sound frequencies that can transform deep-seated fears, allergies, traumas and mental/emotional blocks into useful opportunities of growth and inspiration within a matter of moments. Andreas's latest system "Art of Self-Healing" (as Book/CD or DVD), to be released at the end of 2006, is comprised of his Ener-chi Art and specific Sacred Santémony sounds.

John Hornecker

Each of us must find our own path in life, but if we are fortunate we will encounter mentors along the way who show us new possibilities. I am grateful to acknowledge that I have had more than my share, with Andreas Moritz being an important one of them.

I was born in 1936, and grew up on a small farm in Oregon. Our large family garden and orchard provided an abundance of healthy vegetables, berries and fruits. We also raised a few farm animals to provide meat, eggs and milk. As I left the farm and migrated to a cosmopolitan life, I gravitated toward some of the careless eating and lifestyle habits all too common among my contemporaries. However, starting in1970, I experienced a spiritual awakening, became a vegetarian, and also stopped drinking coffee, alcohol and other unhealthy beverages.

With these shifts in consciousness, diet and lifestyle, and by educating myself about natural approaches to health through innumerable workshops and books, I have enjoyed a life of excellent health and vitality for the past 35 years. However, as I found myself progressing toward my 'senior' years, I realized that I was still buying into the cultural mindset that says as we advance in age, we can expect a general decline in our state of health.

I met Andreas Moritz in 1998 at a peace conference in Israel. His incredible understanding of the human body and how it functions has opened a world of new possibilities to me – a world that enables continued health and vitality regardless of age. From Andreas I have learn that deteriorating health is most often caused by the gradual accumulation of residues in our vital organs, which inhibit them from doing their important jobs. Through relatively simple internal cleansing processes, we can restore the normal healthy functioning of our organs, and enjoy continued health and vitality throughout our life.

Andreas has written a series of comprehensive books on health, nutrition and lifestyle that can be of great assistance to all of us – they certainly have been to me. But the extensive amount of information can be a bit overwhelming for someone who may be just starting to move toward a more natural approach to health. So I have been grateful for the opportunity to collaborate with Andreas in creating this introductory book. It is intended to provide basic information that will enable you to make more enlightened life decisions related to your personal health and well-being.

John

OTHER BOOKS, PRODUCTS AND SERVICES BY ANDREAS MORITZ

The Amazing Liver and Gallbladder Flush

In this revised edition of his best-selling book, *The Amazing Liver Cleanse,* Andreas Moritz addresses the most common but rarely recognized cause of illness – gallstones congesting the liver. This book provides a thorough understanding of what causes gallstones in the liver and gallbladder and provides the reader with do-it-yourself instructions to painlessly remove them in the comfort of one's home. It also gives practical guidelines on how to prevent new gallstones from being formed.

Timeless Secrets of Health & Rejuvenation

This book puts the responsibility of health care back where it belongs – into the hands of every individual. Healing occurs effortlessly and naturally once the body returns to its natural state – perfect balance and utmost efficiency. The author describes the methods for achieving this state of balance regardless of age and previous health problems. *Timeless Secrets of Health & Rejuvenation,* which is a revised and greatly expanded version of his previous book entitled, *The Key to Health and Rejuvenation,* opens the door for everyone to lead a stress-free life and enjoy continued youth and vitality for the rest of one's life.

Cancer Is Not A Disease!
It's A Survival Mechanism

This latest book by Andreas Moritz may rock or even dismantle the very foundation of your beliefs about the body, health and healing. It offers the open-minded reader concerned about cancer a radically different understanding of what cancer really is. According to Andreas Moritz, cancer is a desperate and final attempt by the body to stay alive for as long as circumstances permit – circumstances that are, in fact, in your control.

Today's conventional approaches of killing, cutting or burning cancerous cells offer a mere 7% "success" rate for cancer remission, and the majority of the few survivors are "cured" for just a period of five years or less. In this book, you will discover what actually causes cancer and why it is so important to heal the whole person, not just the symptoms of cancer. You will also learn that cancer occurs only after all other defense mechanisms in the body have failed, for obvious reasons. A malignant tumor is not a vicious monster that is out to kill us in retaliation for our sins or abuse of our body. As you will find out, cancer does not attempt to kill the body; to the contrary, it tries to save it. However, unless we change our perception of what cancer really is, it will continue to threaten the life of one out of every two people. This book opens a door to those who wish to become whole again, in body, mind and spirit.

It's Time to Come Alive

In this book, previously entitled *It's Time to Wake Up*, Andreas Moritz brings to light our deep, inner need for abundance, love and spiritual wisdom. In addition, he assists the reader in developing a new sense of reality that is based on trust, power and happiness. He describes in detail our relationship with the natural world and how we can harness its tremendous powers for our personal benefit, as well as that of humanity as a whole. *It's Time to Come Alive* challenges some of our most ardently held beliefs and offers a way out of the restrictions and limitations we have created in our lives.

Lifting the Veil of Duality

In *Lifting the Veil of Duality,* previously entitled *Freedom from*

Judgment, best-selling author, Andreas Moritz, poignantly exposes the illusion of duality. He outlines a simple way to remove virtually every limitation that you have imposed upon yourself during the course of living duality. You will be invited to see yourself and the world through a new lens – the lens of clarity, discernment and non-judgment. The author suggests that mistakes, accidents, coincidences, negativity, deception, injustice, wars, crime and terrorism all have a deeper purpose and meaning in the larger scheme of things. Although some of these ideas may conflict with the beliefs you currently hold, you are invited to read this book with an open mind, for an open mind is well poised to lift the veil of duality.

Heart Disease No More!
Make Peace with Your Heart and Heal Yourself
(excerpted from Timeless Secrets of Health & Rejuvenation)

Less than one hundred years ago, heart disease was an extremely rare disease. Today it kills more people in the developed world than all other causes of death combined. Despite the vast amount of financial resources spent on finding a cure for heart disease, the current medical approaches remain mainly symptom-oriented and do not address the underlying causes.

Even worse: There is overwhelming evidence to show that the treatment of heart disease or its presumed precursors, such as high blood pressure, hardening of the arteries and high cholesterol, does not only prevent a real cure but can easily lead to chronic heart failure. The patient's heart may still beat, but not strong enough to feel vital and alive.

Without removing the underlying causes of heart disease and its precursors, there is little, if any, protection against it. Heart attacks can strike regardless whether you have had a coronary bypass done or stents placed inside your arteries. According to research, these procedures fail to prevent heart attacks or reduce mortality rates.

Heart Disease No More, excerpted from the author's bestselling Timeless Secrets of Health & Rejuvenation, puts the responsibility for healing where it belongs, that is, to the heart, mind and body of each individual. It provides you with the practical insights about how heart disease develops, what causes it and what you can do to prevent and reverse it for good, regardless of a possible genetic predisposition.

Art of Self-Healing
Instantly Access The Power
To Heal Your Body, Mind and Emotions!
(Available end of 2006)

At this time of great challenge and confusion in all areas of life – individual, social, national and international – we are also blessed with powerful solutions to our most pressing problems. Something we least expected, art and sound are now emerging to become the leading healing methods of our time.

Art of Self-Healing by bestselling author and health practitioner, Andreas Moritz, is a unique approach that gives a person instant access to his/her own healing powers. The approach consists of a series of 32 light-ray-imbued pictures (Ener-Chi Art) created by the author, and specific healing sounds (Sacred Santémony) that he has recorded on CD for the purpose of removing any obstacles to healing one's body and mind and emotions. The supplied CD is synchronized with viewing the pictures for about half a minute each.

All books are available as paperback copies and electronic books (except Art of Self-Healing) from the Ener-Chi Wellness Center.

Website: http://www.ener-chi.com
Email: Enerchiart@aol.com

Phone: (864) 848 6410 or (615) 676-9961

Sacred Santémony –
for Emotional Healing

Sacred Santémony is a unique healing system that uses sounds from specific words to balance deep emotional/spiritual imbalances. The powerful words produced in Sacred Santémony are made from whole-brain use of the letters of the *ancient language* – language that is comprised of the basic sounds that underlie and bring forth all physical manifestation. The letters of the ancient language vibrate at a much higher level than our modern languages, and when combined to form whole words, they generate feelings of peace and harmony (Santémony) to calm the storms of unrest, violence and turmoil, both internal and external.

In April 2002, I spontaneously began to chant sounds that are meant to improve certain health conditions. These sounds resembled chants by Native Americans, Tibetan monks, Vedic pundits (Sanskrit) and languages from other star systems (not known on planet Earth). Within two weeks, I was able to bring forth sounds that would instantly remove emotional blocks and resistance or aversion to certain situations and people, foods, chemicals, thought forms, beliefs, etc. The following are but a few examples of what Sacred Santémony is able to assist you with:

- Reducing or removing fear that is related to death, disease, the body, foods, harmful chemicals, parents and other people, lack of abundance, impoverishment, phobias, environment-al threats, the future and the past, unstable economic trends, political unrest, etc.
- Clearing or reducing a recent or current hurt, disappointment or anger resulting from past emotional trauma or negative experiences in life.
- Cleansing of the *Akashic Records* (a recording of all experiences the soul has gathered throughout all life streams) from persistent fearful elements, including the

idea and concept that we are separate from and not one with Spirit, God or our Higher Self.

- Setting the preconditions for you to resolve your karmic issues not through pain and suffering, but through creativity and joy.
- Improving or clearing up allergies and intolerances to foods, chemical substances, pesticides, herbicides, air pollutants, radiation, medical drugs, pharmaceutical byproducts, etc.
- Undoing the psycho-emotional root causes of any chronic illness, including cancer, heart disease, MS, diabetes, arthritis, brain disorders, depression, etc.
- Resolving other difficulties or barriers in life by "converting" them into the useful blessings that they really are.

To arrange for a personal Sacred Santémony session with Andreas Moritz, please follow the same directions as given for Telephone Consultations.
(As of 2006, the fee for a half hour is $85)

Ener-Chi Art

Andreas Moritz has developed a new system of healing and rejuvenation designed to restore the basic life energy (Chi) of an organ or a system in the body within a matter of seconds. Simultaneously, it also helps balance the emotional causes of illness.

Eastern approaches to healing, such as Acupuncture and Shiatsu, are intended to enhance well-being by stimulating and balancing the flow of Chi to the various organs and systems of the body. In a similar manner, the energetics of Ener-Chi Art is designed to restore a balanced flow of Chi throughout the body.

According to most ancient systems of health and healing, the balanced flow of Chi is the key determinant for a healthy body and mind. When Chi flows through the body unhindered, health and vitality are maintained. By contrast, if the flow of Chi is disrupted or reduced, health and vitality tend to decline.

A person can determine the degree to which the flow of Chi is balanced in the body's organs and systems by using a simple muscle testing procedure. To reveal the effectiveness of Ener-Chi Art, it is important to apply this test both before and after viewing each Ener-Chi Art picture.

To allow for easy application of this system, Andreas has created a number of healing paintings that have been "activated" through a unique procedure that imbues each work of art with specific color rays (derived from the higher dimensions). To receive the full benefit of an Ener-Chi Art picture all that is necessary is to look at it for less than a minute. During this time, the flow of Chi within the organ or system becomes fully restored. When applied to all the organs and systems of the body, Ener-Chi Art sets the precondition for the whole body to heal and rejuvenate itself.

Ener-Chi Ionized Stones

Ener-Chi Ionized Stones are stones and crystals that have been energized, activated, and imbued with life force through a special activation process introduced by Andreas Moritz – the founder of Ener-Chi Art.

Stone ionization has not been attempted before because stones and rocks have rarely been considered useful in the field of healing. Yet, stones have the inherent power to hold and release vast amounts of information and energy. Once ionized, they exert a balancing influence on everything with which they come into contact. The ionization of stones may be one of our keys to survival in a world that is experiencing high-level pollution and destruction of its eco-balancing systems.

In the early evolutionary stages of Earth, every particle of matter within the mantle of the planet contained within it the blueprint of the entire planet, just as every cell of our body contains within its DNA structure the blueprint of our entire body. The blueprint information within every particle of matter is still there – it has simply fallen into a dormant state. The ionization process "reawakens" this original blueprint information, and enables the associated energies to be released. In this sense, Ener-Chi Ionized Stones are alive and conscious, and are able to energize, purify and balance any natural substance with which they come into contact.

By placing an Ionized Stone next to a glass of water or plate of food, the water or food becomes energized, thereby increasing digestibility and nutrient absorption. Ionized stones can also be used effectively in conjunction with Ener-Chi Art – simply place an Ionized Stone on the corresponding area of the body while viewing an Ener-Chi Art picture. For more potential uses please check out the web site given below.

Telephone Consultations
For a Personal Telephone Consultation with Andreas Moritz, please

1. Call or send an email with your name, phone number, address, digital picture (if you have one) of your face and any other relevant information to Andreas.

2. Set up an appointment for the length of time you choose to spend with him. A comprehensive consultation lasts 2 hours or more. Shorter consultations deal with all the questions you may have and the information that is relevant to your specific health issue(s).

Fees (2005/06): $85 for 1/2 hour, $170 for one hour, $255 for 1 1/2 hours, and $340 for 2 hours

Note: Shorter consultations deal with all the questions you may have and the information that is relevant to your specific health issue(s). For a comprehensive consultation, (if you have a digital camera) please take a snapshot of your face (preferably without makeup) and email it to Andreas before your appointment with him. This can greatly assist Andreas in assisting you in your quest for better health.

To order Ener-chi Art pictures, Ionized Stones and other products
please contact:

Ener-Chi Wellness Center, LLC
Web Site: http://www.ener-chi.com
E-mail: enerchiart@aol.com

Phone: (864) 848-6410 (USA)
E-voice: (615) 676-9961 (USA)

Lightning Source UK Ltd.
Milton Keynes UK
UKHW010731130123
415295UK00001B/80